Middle Ear Implant: Implantable Hearing Aids

Advances in Audiology

Vol. 4

Series Editor
M. Hoke, Münster

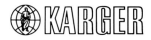 KARGER

Basel · München · Paris · London · New York · New Delhi · Singapore · Tokyo · Sydney

Middle Ear Implant: Implantable Hearing Aids

Volume Editor
J.-I. Suzuki, Tokyo

117 figures and 19 tables, 1988

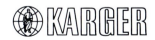 KARGER

Basel · München · Paris · London · New York · New Delhi · Singapore · Tokyo · Sydney

Advances in Audiology

Contents

Contents

Human Application

Acknowledgment

The authors extend their thanks to Mrs. Chizuko Umezawa, Agency
of Industry, Science and Technology, for her valuable suggestions related
to this publication, and also to Miss Hiroko Banno and Tomoko Yoko-
yama for their excellent secretarial work.

Preface

For the hearing-impaired, to improve their ability to hear by means of an implanted hearing aid has been a long-cherished dream. At last, their desire has started to look more attainable during the past ten or so years, a time when existing hearing aids began to be miniaturized and their quality remarkably improved.

An implantable hearing aid has always been a desired goal for otologists, audiologists, and engineers as well. With the development of the behind-the-ear type hearing device, which was soon to be followed by the appearance of the in-the-ear type, the latter extremely small, the chances for perfecting an implantable hearing aid became a real possibility.

Still, to turn an implantable hearing aid into reality required many issues to be discussed by those who were capable of bringing such a device about, experts from the fields of medicine and technology. Thus the year 1978 marked the start of a five-year project towards realizing a middle ear implantable hearing aid, this research being funded by a grant-in-aid from the Japanese government.

Although the authors have used more or less different terms in their previous papers on implanted hearing aids, the new device should now have an appropriate terminology. As it is implanted in the middle ear to act as a hearing aid, the term 'middle ear implantable hearing aid' is literally explanatory. At the time of this publication, we decided to use 'middle ear implant' (MEI). 'Middle ear implant' is related to 'cochlear implant', a widely used term meaning 'cochlear implantable hearing aid'. Totally implantable and partially implantable types of MEI may be abbreviated as total MEI or T-MEI and partial MEI or P-MEI, respectively.

The year 1978 was an auspicious time to begin. Great technological advancements were being made in fields that would provide support – electronics, biocompatible materials, developing technology of artificial organs, microsurgical techniques in otology, as well other related areas. Good cooperation, however, was essential for success. Without this, decisions might not have been appropriate and difficulties not overcome. Fortunately, the Agency of Industrial Science and Technology (AIST), under the auspices of the Ministry of International Trade and Industry, launched this endeavor at an opportune time and under exceptional circumstances. Experts from these various fields were able to work together closely for a period of five years. AIST then selected two firms – Rion Co., Ltd. and Sanyo Electric Co., Ltd. – to accomplish this project and, at the same time, organized an Advisory Committee to assist and monitor their progress. Members of this committee consisted of authorities in technology, electronics, energy sources, acoustics, otology, audiology, and rehabilitation, as may be seen in the list at the end of the Preface.

The committee exerted every effort towards guiding the project to its ultimate success. This was not easy. There were important, critical decisions that had to be made, which animal experiments were to be undertaken, other considerations being the implantation of a miniature microphone under the skin, and identifying the function of the ceramic bimorph, which was proposed by this committee as the only useful vibrator.

The animal experiments were successfully performed, their good results proving largely dependent on the use of auditory brainstem-evoked responses in evaluating the hearing acuity in cats. In these experiments the use of auditory brainstem-evoked responses showed itself to be a reliable and efficient tool.

The project was terminated successfully in March 1983. At this time, the medical and rehabilitation team began to apply the project product to selected patients. Our success, which has been well received both by the public and the experts in and outside of our country, should now be extended to broader use.

Since 1983, our efforts have focussed on clinical application. Slowly, but steadily, we have accumulated data on cases who are being carefully monitored with follow-ups. Fortunately, our Ministry of Health and Welfare has left the supervision of the clinical application of the MEI in the hands of the previous Advisory Committee.

At this important stage of MEI development, Prof. M. Hoke, Chief Editor of *Advances in Audiology,* published by S. Karger, suggested that we compile a book on our research to be published by his company. His kind advice has been accepted.

We should like to take this opportunity to express our gratitude to Profs R. L. Goode, A. Tjellström and Mr. J. Heide and to the members of their teams, who so generously accepted our invitation to be included among the authors of this book. We would also like to extend our thanks to Dr. T. Karger, Chairman, and Ms. D. Greder of S. Karger AG, Basel, and to Mr. H. Katakura, President of Katakura Libri, Inc., for their kind cooperation in insuring the success of this publication.

December, 1987   *Jun-Ichi Suzuki, MD*

Development Committee of MEI of Japan (1978–1983)

Jun-Ichi Suzuki	Teikyo University School of Medicine, Chairman of the committee and also chairman of the subcommittee for experimental evaluation
Naoaki Yanagihara	Ehime University School of Medicine, Chairman of the subcommittee for clinical evaluation
Taichiro Akiyama	Japan Biomedical Material Research Center
Sotaro Funasaka	The University of Tokyo, Branch Hospital, for the year 1978
Yukio Inukai	Industrial Products Research Institute, Agency of Industrial Science and Technology, for the years 1978–1980
Keijiro Koga	National Childrens' Hospital
Nagamasa Sakabe	Central Hospital of Japanese National Railways
Minoru Toriyama	National Medical Center Hospital
Shizuo Hiki	Research Center for Applied Information Sciences, Tohoku University
Toshiki Manabe	National Rehabilitation Center for the Disabled
Hajime Miura	Electrotechnical Laboratory, Agency of Industrial Science and Technology
Shiro Yoshizawa	Faculty of Engineering, Kyoto University
Hisao Shono	Rion Co., Ltd.
Hironosuke Ikeda	Sanyo Electric Co., Ltd.

History and Principle

Adv. Audiol., vol. 4, pp. 1–14 (Karger, Basel 1988)

Early Studies and the History of Development of the Middle Ear Implant in Japan

Jun-Ichi Suzuki[a], *Hisao Shono*[b], *Keijiro Koga*[c], *Taichiro Akiyama*[d]

[a] Department of Otolaryngology, Teikyo University School of Medicine;
[b] Rion Co., Ltd., Tokyo; [c] National Childrens' Hospital, Tokyo; [d] Japan Biomedical Material Research Center, Tokyo, Japan

Over the years, hearing aids have appeared to be different in many ways from visual aids or eyeglasses, which have been widely accepted as useful and even as attractive accessories. Nonetheless, hearing aids have been helpful for hearing-impaired people, although their benefits have been limited to only a small percentage of users, and satisfaction with them has frequently fallen far below expectations.

Hearing aids have given the impression that their users are handicapped [Blood, 1977]. Accordingly, moderately or lightly hearing-impaired individuals often shunned their use and hoped for a device that would not be visible to other people. Due to remarkable improvements in their function and a reduction in size, hearing aids have gradually become more popular and acceptable to an increasing majority.

The dream of implanting a miniature hearing aid, a hope long cherished by every hearing-impaired, has recently become a reality [Watanabe, 1965; Goode, 1970, 1975, 1977; Vernon et al., 1972; Vernon, 1976; Glorig et al., 1972; Fredrickson et al., 1973; Cook et al., 1973; Northern, 1973; Nunley et al., 1976].

Background for the Development of the Middle Ear Implant or
Implantable Hearing Aid

Hearing Aids: Successful Miniaturization and
Sophistication in Function
It was in 1900 that F. Alt in Austria first developed an electronic hearing aid using a carbon microphone. In 1902, in America, M. R.

	1974	1975	1976	1977	1978	1979	1980	1981	1982	1983	1984	1985
Eyeglass	108.7	89.4	74.6	43.3	56.4	46.3	39.3	37.6	32.1	27.9	17.5	12.8
Body-worn	35.3	30.3	22.0	12.0	22.5	21.0	20.3	16.3	15.1	12.5	9.2	10.5
ITE	21.6	64.7	104.2	132.8	174.0	193.9	248.7	315.3	359.0	508.7	646.7	746.3
BTE	335.9	355.9	295.3	222.5	332.1	379.1	428.3	465.0	448.3	480.6	437.6	383.9
All types	501.6	540.4	496.1	410.6	585.1	640.3	736.6	834.2	854.5	1029.7	1110.9	1153.6

ITE = In-the-ear type. BTE = Behind-the-ear type.

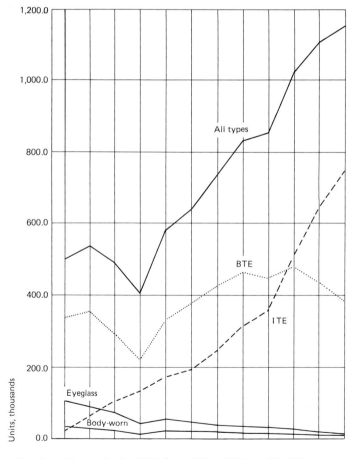

Fig. 1. Hearing aid sales in the USA from 1974–1985 [modified from Mahon, 1985].

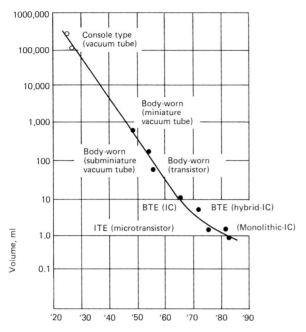

Fig. 2. Changes in typical hearing aid size. ○ = American aid; ● = Japanese aid. BTE = behind-the-ear type; ITE = in-the-ear type; IC = induction coil [modified from Shono, 1984].

Hatchinson started to produce the 'Akouphon', also using a carbon microphone, on a commercial basis. In 1904, in Denmark, H. Demant established a company to distribute American aids 'Acousticon' and 'Akustic'. In 1940, W. Demant, his son, began manufacturing their own aids, and this company was later called 'Oticon'. Phonophor Corp. subsidiary of Siemens, which started to produce hearing aids 'Phonophor' in 1908, has been very important in the history of this device [Berger, 1970].

Miniaturization, started with the transistor in 1952, was accelerated with the induction coil in 1964. Subsequently, in 1965, Zenith introduced the 'in-the-ear type' hearing aid. Figure 1 shows the changes in the types of hearing aids used over the last 12 years in the United States.

Miniaturization of hearing aids was parallel to functional improvement. Fitting of hearing aids is necessary and requires expert help to be successful. Thus, moderately hearing-impaired people have come to find these modern hearing aids useful for daily conversation when they are properly adjusted to the patient's specific disability. Figure 2 shows the remarkable reduction in the size of hearing aids achieved since 1924.

Otomicrosurgery: More Success with Tympanoplasty and
Stapedectomy as a Preparation for the Implantation of the
Implantable Hearing Aid, or Middle Ear Implant

Tympanoplasty is mostly applied to chronically infected ears, while stapedectomy is generally performed in those with no infections. Because of this, the use of artificial materials has been successful in stapes surgery. And, in tympanoplasty for chronic otitis media, many surgeons are very, very careful in using artificial ossicles.

Some parts of the middle ear implant (MEI) have to be implanted in the middle ear cavity, although most parts are placed under the skin, in the soft tissues and on the bone. Otomicrosurgical techniques, based on various experiences over the last 30 years, have turned out to be very useful for the MEI project.

As long as the MEI has maximum biocompatibility and continues to function under the very severe conditions of 100% salty humidity, that is, as long as its medical function is assured, surgeons need have little worry about the implanting technique itself. In other words, surgical techniques to implant a foreign body under the skin in and around the temporal bone have been sufficiently developed, and success can be close to 100% if there is no infection present.

Implantable Artificial Organs: Experiences and Development in Other
Medical Fields and Electrical and Biological Housing

The MEI is certainly one of the most exciting artificial organs in medicine today. Remarkable developments in both basic technology, especially in biomedical materials and electronics, and in basic medical and surgical sciences are the bedrock of its development. Without basic research in biocompatibility and without scientific research in medical function, the present MEI would have been inconceivable, and there would be no possibility of final success. Furthermore, it must be said that there are a number of negative feelings and opinions concerning artificial organs, especially when they are to be implanted in the body. All types of risk have to be considered. In particular, with such a delicate instrument as a hearing aid, the high possibility of breakdown or deterioration must be borne in mind. The best technology, needless to say, must be used, but still, a wide variety of safety mechanisms with an equally wide variety of functions must be employed.

The MEI project would not have been feasible if it had been proposed 5 years earlier than it was. It was, in fact, launched at precisely the right time from many standpoints: high-polymer chemistry, biocompatibility research, electronic technology, medical engineering, surgical technology, and so on. Thus, in the 5 years since 1978, the MEI has crystallized as the best technology in Japan.

Diagnostic Hearing Examinations: Progress and Sophistication

Hearing examinations are making the best use of modern developments in electronic technology. This sophistication in clinical and experimental hearing tests may be difficult to find in other areas of medicine and, in fact, is probably comparable to the level extant in ophthalmology.

E. P. Fowler, R. L. Wegel and H. Fletcher in America reported the first clinically useful audiometer and recommended the audiogram that we are using today. The Békésy type audiometer was introduced in 1947, and ASA regulations on audiometers were set in 1951, an indication that this device was in wide use by then. Following this, the advent of computers brought about many changes in hearing tests. Thus, cochleograms (1967) and the auditory brainstem response (ABR, 1970) have come to be important objective examinations useful in both human and animal experiments.

Over the years, then, sophisticated hearing tests have become available and certainly indispensable in determining the exact indications for the MEI, as demonstrated later in this work. Objective audiometry, especially the ABR, was applied to animal experiments in the present MEI project, and substantially shortened the term of the basic research. The usefulness, reproducibility and easy applicability of the ABR were maximally taken advantage of during the experiments.

Initial Discussions and Conclusions for Developing the MEI

Certainly before the 5-year project was started, there were heated discussions as to what the MEI was supposed to be. And these discussions were the basis on which the Agency of Industrial Science and Technology (AIST) selected this as a government-aided project in 1983.

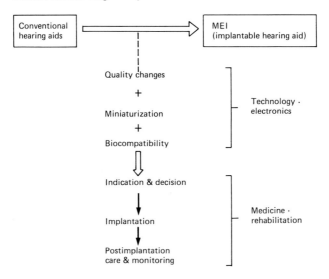

Fig. 3. Aiming at the implantation of hearing aids.

There were several basic expectations or requirements for the project proposals to be accepted, namely, the following:

(1) Social needs for the project have to be strong and urgent.

(2) The techniques and products have to be entirely new, at least in our country.

(3) The techniques and products have to be extremely useful for medicine and rehabilitation.

(4) The techniques and products are expected to reduce medical and rehabilitation expenditures.

The limiting conditions for the project proposals to be accepted are as follows:

(1) The research and development (R and D) alone may require from 100 million to 1,000 million yen.

(2) There is some possibility that the R and D may terminate in failure.

(3) The R and D may require intensive teamwork by experts in different fields, for example, technology, medicine and rehabilitation, from both the public and private sector.

(4) The R and D is on a leading level worldwide and will have a strong halo effect on related R and D. The R and D has to be accepted for wide utilization by the Ministry of Health and Welfare.

In order to make the project proposal practical and useful, it had to be shown that the R and D target is clearly attainable within 3–5 years, namely, that sufficient basic research has been previously accomplished. In addition, the risks of failure have to be moderate, neither too high, nor too low.

Thus, the MEI project was accepted by AIST in 1973 as the above-mentioned conditions and requirements were then considered reasonably fulfilled. In spite of the many favorable discussions about the project proposals for the MEI, there were many necessary steps to be taken, as shown in figure 3. So the first of the 5 years of the MEI project was taken up with continuing the previous discussions. The conclusions about the basic structure of the MEI were as follows.

Energy Source: Partial and Total Implantation of the MEI

The matter of the energy source was another subject of long and repeated discussions, which do not appear to have ended even now. This is because we do not feel satisfied with our present solution.

In the course of our discussions on the energy supply, we decided to produce two types of MEI, totally implantable (T-MEI) and partially implantable (P-MEI) (fig. 4). Considerations as to the energy source were to be made only for the former type, since in the latter type, only driving signals would be supplied through the skin from the external part of the MEI. Although we can expect even better energy sources in the not-too-distant future, the conclusions reached by the advisory committee in 1978–1979 were as follows:

(1) The totally implantable MEI is to be supplied by a nonrechargeable primary lithium-manganese battery, or a secondary rechargeable nickel-cadmium battery.

(2) The partially implantable MEI is to be supplied signals through induction coils to the internal parts of the device. A battery of any kind can be put in the external part.

The size of the MEI was initially expected to be as small as 1 cm³. Although the amplifier and microphone were quite small, the batteries, both the larger primary and the smaller secondary, are relatively large, as can be seen in the figures.

Since the amplifier-battery complex has to be so heavily shielded, both electrically and biologically, it became much larger than initially expected. This complex is to be implanted in the area behind the ear. The internal induction coil for the partially implantable MEI is also to be im-

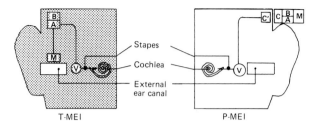

Fig. 4. T-MEI and P-MEI. M = Microphone; A = amplifier; B = battery; V = vibrator; C, C' = external and internal induction coils.

planted in a similar area. The microphone is to be set in the bony external ear canal, and the vibrator-holder should be in the attic-antrum, anchored to the cortex of the temporal bone.

Vibrator: Piezoelectric, but not Electromagnetic

The decision about the vibrator to the stapes was the real key to the project. Repeated discussions, data collection and experiments were necessary. Comparison of the vibrator candidates for the MEI is shown in figure 5. At that stage of technological development, there were two such candidates: the electromagnetic coil and the ceramic bimorph.

Based on the following comparisons, it was finally decided to adopt the ceramic bimorph.

(1) Electroacoustic functions: frequency range, distortions, energy consumption, maximum output, driving power, transient characteristics.

(2) Mechanical characteristics: size, shape, complexity, weight, fragility, durability.

(3) Reliability and safety: interactions with the body and various things outside the body, harmfulness, stability.

The final successful outcome of the MEI project can be directly attributed to this decision. The details of the reasons for this decision are given in part II, Technical Aspects. In short, the ceramic bimorph was considered to be the closest to the ideal vibrator: its functions are independent and stable in the human body and the sound transmissions give high fidelity with little noise. Nonetheless, we wanted a little more power in the output, a little less fragility, and so on. Later, fortunately, it was shown that the sound transmitted by the MEI using the ceramic bimorph was perceived as pure and clear by the subjects using the device.

Type of vibrator		Electro-magnetic		Moving-coil	Piezo-electric
		un-balanced	balanced		
Driving method to the stapes		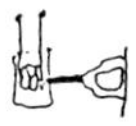	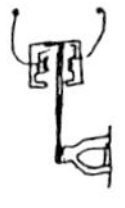	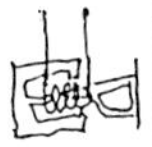	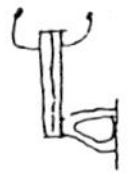
Reliability & safety	deterioration	△	△	●	○
	effect of magnetic induction	△	△	●	+
	easy installation	○	△	●	○
	burden to stapes	○	○	△	○
Electro-acoustic characteristics	frequency characteristics	△	△	●	○
	distortion	●	△	○	+
	energy consumtion	○	+	○	+
	maximum output displacement	○	+	○	△
	driving power	○	○	△	△
	transient characteristics	●	△	○	+
Mechanical characteristics	mechanical strength	△	●	●	△
	shock resistance	●	●	△	△
	moisture resistance	△	△	●	○
Structure	Simplicity	△	●	●	+
	Small size	●	△	●	+
	Light weight	●	△	●	+

Fig. 5. Comparison of the candidates for MEI vibrator. +, ○, △, and ● indicate the expectations, best, good, bad, and worst, respectively.

Microphone: To Be Covered by the Skin

Ultraminiature electret condenser microphones are available. They can be so small as to be installed in the ear-canal-type hearing aid. But the questions to be answered were:

(1) Will the microphones function under the skin?

(2) Will they supply signals strong enough to drive the ceramic bimorph?

The answer to the first question was a matter of housing and electrical and biological shieldings. The second required animal experiments, which, fortunately, gave us positive answers and pushed the MEI project even further forward.

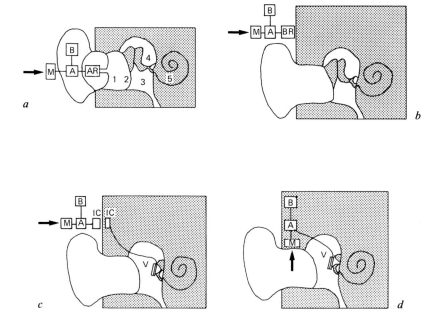

Fig. 6. Comparison of hearing aids. 1 = external auditory canal; 2 = tympanic membrane; 3 = middle ear cavity; 4 = stapes; 5 = inner ear; M = microphone; A = amplifier; AR = air conduction receiver; B = battery; BR = bone conduction receiver; IC = induction coil; V = vibrator. *a* Conventional air-conduction hearing aid. *b* Bone conduction hearing aid. *c* P-MEI. *d* T-MEI.

Comparison of the Proposed Middle Ear Implants and Conventional Hearing Aids

The differences between conventional hearing aids and the proposed middle ear implants are an interesting subject in themselves. Figure 6 shows an air-conduction hearing aid, a bone-conduction hearing aid, a P-MEI and a T-MEI. As can be seen, the differences among them are remarkable, at least from the following standpoints:

(1) Sounds go into the inner ear through the stapes-oval window with both types of MEI and the air-conduction hearing aid. With the bone-conduction hearing aid, the whole skull is vibrated, and the sound signals reach the inner ear. Energy consumption for sound transmission to the inner ear is the least with the MEIs, more with the air-conduction hearing aid and the most with the bone-conduction hearing aid.

(2) There is air vibration for the amplified sound to reach the inner ear with the air-conduction hearing aid, but not with the bone-conduction hearing aid or with either type of MEI. Thus, the transmitted sound has more chance of being distorted with the conventional type of air-conduction hearing aid. The details are shown in part III, Experimental Assessment.

(3) With the exception of the T-MEI, the microphone, amplifier and battery remain outside of the body and can be changed or checked whenever needed. This difference gives rise to both good and bad features in the two types of MEIs.

R and D of the MEI with Governmental Support in Japan

Organization

Governmental support to manufacturing companies was undertaken under the auspices of AIST, one of the family of 12 research institutes belonging to the Ministry of International Trade and Industry (MITI) starting in 1952. In April 1976, AIST inaugurated the National Research and Development Program for Medical and Welfare Apparatus (fig. 7).

The basic principle of the R and D project was to nominate two or more manufacturers and then to fund them to reach a specific goal in a limited number of years. To this end, AIST would organize an advisory committee consisting of medical, rehabilitational and technological experts.

The 5-Year Project for Developing the MEI

Following the system proposed by AIST in 1982, R and D has been completed in five medical projects and in four welfare equipment technology. Ongoing R and D includes three medical and five welfare themes, to which the MEI project belonged. In 1978, two manufacturing companies were nominated to conduct the 5-year project: Rion Company, to develop the hearing aids to be implanted, and Sanyo Electric Company, to develop the battery as an energy source, also to be implanted. The advisory committee, as stated in the Preface, was then organized.

The animal experiments, aimed at testing the microphone, vibrator and the whole MEI in particular, were mainly conducted in cats [Araki et al., 1981; Kodera et al., 1981 a, b; Araki et al., 1983]. ABR was used as a most useful and efficient test to evaluate the hearing in cats before and after MEI implantation. Without ABR, the experiments would have

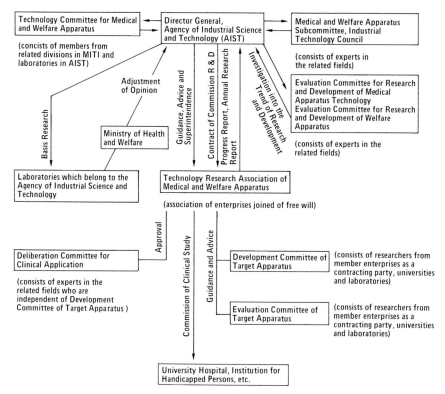

Fig. 7. National Research and Development Program for Medical and Welfare Apparatus in Japan. The scheme is to be effective as a function of the Ministry of International Trade and Industry (MITI).

taken so long that it would not have been possible to complete the project within 5 years or so.

In the middle of the 5-year project, the advisory committee organized two subcommittees, one for experimental evaluation and the other for clinical evaluation.

The subcommittee for experimental evaluation was chaired by J. Suzuki, and the animal experiments were conducted mainly at Teikyo University, as well as at the National Medical Center Hospital, where M. Toriyama was responsible. The subcommittee for clinical evaluation was chaired by N. Yanagihara, and clinical evaluation was conducted at both Ehime University Hospital and Teikyo University Hospital. The details are reported below [Gyo et al., 1982; Yanagihara et al., 1983].

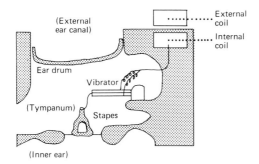

Fig. 8. P-MEI.

The 5-year project ended with success in 1983, and two types of implantable hearing aids or MEI (T-MEI or P-MEI) were developed [Fukuyama et al., 1983; Shono et al., 1983; Ohno, 1984, 1985]. The T-MEI can use either one of the two types of battery, rechargeable and nonrechargeable, while the P-MEI obtains energy from a button cell battery which is contained in the outer part of the MEI and signals fed through the skin using induction coils. The details of this will be described in part II.

Clinical Application of the MEI since 1983

Towards the end of the project, 1983, the Deliberation Committee for Clinical Application chaired by Dr. Masamitsu Oshima examined the product and gave its approval for experimental application of the MEI to clinical cases.

In 1983, the Ministry of Health and Welfare took over this project to support the clinical application of the MEI as extensively as possible. The AIST advisory committee members have continued to serve in the new committee organized by the Ministry of Welfare. This new committee follows up patients implanted with the MEI. The number of implantations was kept small, and careful observations, which were supposed to be reported to the committee and the manufacturers, were made mandatory.

Implantation techniques also have to be standardized for wider use in the future. Two members of the committee, Drs. Yanagihara and Suzuki, have each organized project groups and have both been engaged in implantation. In addition, indications for implantation have to be carefully studied and standardized. The P-MEI (fig. 8) was selected for the first series of trials, as presented in the last part of this book, while the T-MEI will be reported on later.

Both Rion and Sanyo have been carefully observing the outcome and the follow-up results. These companies are now conducting research on mass production of the MEI in order to meet requests from abroad as well as from our own country.

Jun-Ichi Suzuki, MD, Department of Otolaryngology,
Teikyo University School of Medicine, Itabashi-ku, Tokyo (Japan)

Adv. Audiol., vol. 4, pp. 15–21 (Karger, Basel 1988)

Principle, Construction and Indication of the Middle Ear Implant

Jun-Ichi Suzuki^a, Naoaki Yanagihara^b, Minoru Toriyama^c, Nagamasa Sakabe^d

^{a} Department of Otolaryngology, Teikyo University School of Medicine, Tokyo; ^{b} Department of Otolaryngology, Ehime University School of Medicine, Ehime; ^{c} National Medical Center Hospital, Tokyo; ^{d} Japanese National Railways of Central Hospital, Tokyo, Japan

Totally Implantable MEI and Partially Implantable MEI

As reported in the last section, the 5-year project for developing the middle ear implant (MEI) was successfully terminated in 1983. The principle, the construction, the performance and then the theoretical indication of the MEI will just be outlined here; a more detailed description will be given in the following parts.

The totally implantable (T-MEI) and the partially implantable (P-MEI) types of the MEI developed in 1983 are schematically illustrated in figure 1. In the T-MEI, the microphone is implanted under the skin in the external ear canal wall, the amplifier-battery complex, behind the ear, and the vibrator in the tympanum to be attached to the head of the stapes. In the P-MEI, only the internal induction coil and the vibrator are implanted, while the microphone, the battery-amplifier, and the external induction coil are installed in a capsule to be attached outside, on the skin, behind the helix of the ear. Figure 2 presents a more realistic illustration of these two types of the MEI.

Those parts to be implanted are electrically and also biologically shielded in order to be biocompatible, i.e., to have no biological rejections or tissue reactions.

For the T-MEI there are two types of batteries, a primary nonrechargeable lithium-manganese battery and a secondary rechargeable nickel-cadmium battery. The primary battery is designed to continue

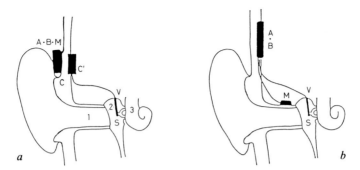

Fig. 1. Two types of implantable MEI. A = Amplifier; B = battery; C, C' = external and internal induction coils; M = microphone; V = vibrator; S = stapes; 1 = external ear canal; 2 = middle ear; 3 = inner ear. *a* Partially implantable MEI. *b* Totally implantable MEI.

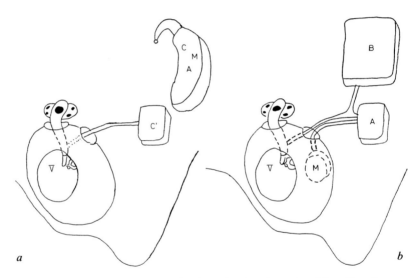

Fig. 2. Schematic illustration of implanted MEI. A = Amplifier; B = battery; C, C' = external and internal induction coils; M = microphone; V = vibrator. *a* Partially implantable MEI. *b* Totally implantable MEI.

working for 2 years and then to be replaced by a new one every 2 years. The secondary battery is recharged through the skin every 2 weeks.

The vibrator consists of piezoelectric ceramic bimorph which vibrates according to the voltage changes applied to each of the two ceramic plates which are glued together. There are two different types of vi-

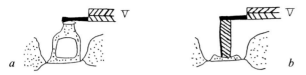

Fig. 3. Connections between the vibrator and the stapes-head *(a)* or the stapes foot plate *(b)*. V = Vibrator, ceramic, bimorph.

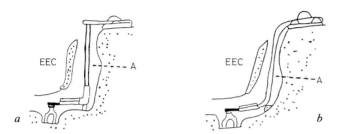

Fig. 4. Two kinds of vibrator holders. These are to be chosen depending on the surgical approach. EEC = External ear canal; A = antrum. *a* The vibrator holder convenient for posterior canal wall-preserving type surgery. *b* The vibrator holder convenient for posterior canal-reconstructing type surgery.

brator, namely, one to be applied to the head of the stapes and the other to the stapes foot plate (fig. 3).

There are also two types of vibrator holders, to be chosen by the surgeon according to the different approaches: one for the ear-canal-preserving surgery and the other for the ear-canal-reconstructive surgery (fig. 4).

The microphone being used is an ultraminiature electret condenser microphone which functions under the skin. The microphone is installed in a hermetically sealed box of medical grade stainless steel with a 9-μm-thick diaphragm and then doubly coated by a biologically inert material, epoxy and parilen.

Performance of the P-MEI and T-MEI

The lowest hearing thresholds after implantation of the P-MEI and the T-MEI in relation to bone-conduction thresholds are shown in figure 5. The thresholds for 4,000 Hz are lower than those for 1,000 Hz by

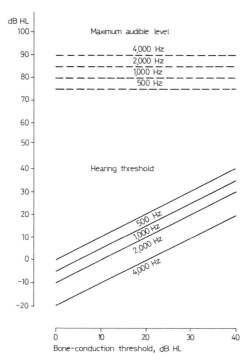

Fig. 5. Hearing threshold and maximum audible level after P-MEI implantation in patients with elevated bone-conduction threshold.

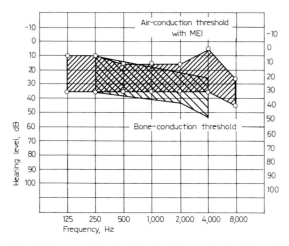

Fig. 6. Bone-conduction threshold as an indication of P-MEI and postimplantation air-conduction threshold.

15–20 dB in either type. The P-MEI type has a lower threshold than the latter by 5–10 dB at all frequencies.

The hearing will show frequency-dependent improvement as shown in figure 6. This figure shows exactly how much air-conduction threshold would be acquired when a normal-hearing individual has his ossicular chain replaced by the MEI, namely, his hearing will be supernormal at higher frequencies.

Indications for MEI Implantation

As mentioned and illustrated above, the MEI exactly replaces the function of the amplification of sound intensity of the normal middle ear. There is greater amplification in higher frequencies, the figure being about 15 dB at the peak (fig. 6). The above data would result in the following indications: The MEI should be indicated for the mixed type deafness with a bone-conduction threshold higher than 30–40 dB in the speech range. When the bone conduction threshold is higher than 40 dB in the speech range, MEI cannot be efficiently used. When the bone conduction threshold is lower than 20 dB in the speech range, and when tympanoplasty cannot be successfully applied, then the MEI may be applied.

In other words, as a principle, tympanoplasty is indicated for the mixed type deafness where the bone-conduction threshold is less than 20 dB, while the MEI is indicated for the mixed type deafness where the bone-conduction threshold is between 20 and 40 dB. Tympanoplasty plus hearing aids are indicated for the mixed type deafness where the bone-conduction threshold is higher than 40 dB (fig. 7).

The best feature of the MEI is that it transmits low-distorted, or high-fidelity sound to the inner ear. The MEI-implanted subjects would enjoy the 'pure', 'clear' and 'less noisy' sounds in contrast to the sounds those subjects used to hear through the hearing aids. Because of this, the above-mentioned indication for MEI – which is restricted theoretically to those with mixed deafness with a bone conduction threshold between 20 and 40 dB – may be extended up and down by 5–10 dB as a relative indication.

The readers are advised to refer to part IV, Human Application, where there are detailed reports on the MEI-implanted cases together with the assessment of audiological and surgical results during the follow-up examinations.

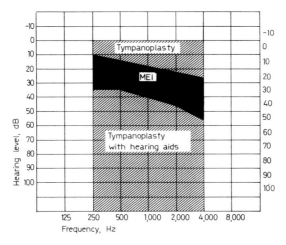

Fig. 7. Indications for tympanoplasty, P-MEI and hearing aids seen from the bone-conduction thresholds.

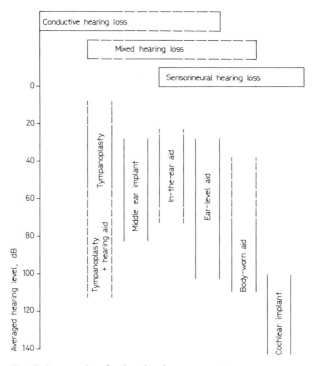

Fig. 8. Approaches for hearing improvement.

When attempting to improve hearing, the first step is to diagnose what kind of hearing impairment one is confronted with. There are three major categories in hearing losses: conductive, mixed and sensorineural hearing losses. There are approaches for improving the hearing losses according to the above three major categories of hearing loss and also according to the degree of hearing loss. The available approaches at this moment are hearing aids of different kinds, tympanoplasty, the combination of tympanoplasty with hearing aids, MEI and cochlear implant. Indications for hearing improvement utilizing the above approaches are shown in figure 8.

Jun-Ichi Suzuki, MD, Department of Otolaryngology,
Teikyo University School of Medicine, Itabashi-ku, Tokyo (Japan)

Adv. Audiol., vol. 4, pp. 22–31 (Karger, Basel 1988)

Electromagnetic Implantable Hearing Aids

Richard L. Goode

Division of Otolaryngology, Department of Surgery, Stanford University
Medical Center, Stanford, Calif., USA

A conventional hearing aid consists of a microphone, an audio frequency amplifier (usually with frequency shaping capability and automatic gain control), a battery and an output transducer, the receiver. An implantable hearing aid may be viewed as an extension of conventional hearing aid technology in that one or more of the hearing aid components are surgically implanted in the ear. Whereas all the components could be implanted, the potential acoustical benefits occur with implantation of only the output transducer, the rest of the components remain external. The indications for an implantable hearing aid for a sensorineural hearing loss are the same as a conventional aid. In this respect, the indications for an implantable hearing aid differ significantly from those for a cochlear implant, since the cochlear implant is designed for profoundly deaf patients who are unable to use a hearing aid. Implantable hearing aids can also be used for conductive losses that cannot be corrected by surgery.

The theoretical acoustic advantage of an implantable aid is that by eliminating the receiver and driving the ossicles directly, there would be an improvement in sound fidelity compared with a conventional hearing aid. The receiver has been shown to be the basis for a portion of the distortion produced by conventional aids [1]. In an aid with the output transducer implanted, the ear canal can be left open, a definite advantage. An open ear canal fitting provides improved speech discrimination in patients with a sloping sensorineural hearing loss compared with closed or partially closed canal fittings [2,3]. Feedback may be a problem in open canal or widely vented fittings at higher gains; an aid with an implantable output stage does not produce acoustic feedback, another potential advantage.

Although a totally implantable aid would provide an invisible prosthesis and perhaps improve patient acceptance, it does not appear to offer any acoustical advantage over implantation of the output stage alone and adds significant technical problems. At this time the technical difficulties of total implantation do not appear to be worth the benefits, which are primarily cosmetic. This chapter, therefore, discusses electromagnetic induction aids in which only the output stage is implanted. We have studied this type of aid in our laboratory since 1969 [4–7].

An implant aid must justify its existence by either providing improved sound reception or increased ease of use when compared with a conventional aid. The implantable component should be nonirritating, trouble free and have a long life expectancy. The surgical procedure used to insert the implantable stage needs to be simple and free of major complications. Ideally it would be performed as an office procedure using local anesthesia. The implant should be easily removable, so that if unsatisfactory it can be removed without incident. The implantable component should not reduce residual hearing when the unit is not energized nor limit activities such as swimming or predispose the patient to recurrent infection. It should not interfere with the wearing of a conventional aid, since under certain circumstances a conventional aid may be indicated. Finally, the externally worn portion of the aid should be similar in size and operating expense to that of conventional ear level aids and its battery drain similar to that of high power ear level aids.

Electromagnetic Induction Hearing

Wilska [8, 9] was apparently the first to use this method to stimulate the middle ear. He placed 'small pieces of soft iron, weighing about 10 mg' on the tympanic membrane of a human subject. Current was delivered by a variable-frequency oscillator to a coil placed over the ear canal. The resulting magnetic field caused the iron and attached tympanic membrane to move so that the subject 'heard' a pure tone. The perceived tone was twice that of the stimulus fequency. This frequency doubling would be expected with an iron particle on the tympanic membrane since the magnetic field produced with each half-cycle of coil current would attract the iron (and eardrum) regardless of the change in field polarity. Thus, the tympanic membrane would be laterally displaced twice for every cycle of stimulating current. By using a superimposed, constant

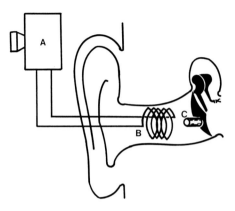

Fig. 1. The principle of the electromagnetic implant hearing aid. See text for details.

magnetic field, Wilska could eliminate the doubling effect; however, the strong magnetic attraction caused 'discomfort and pain'. Wilska also attached a small 1×3 mm coil to the tympanic membrane and placed the ear in a strong, constant magnetic field. When a sinusoidal current was sent into the coil, 'excellent tone' was perceived, but the coil temperature caused burning and pain. Wilska summarized his experiments by stating, 'The essential feature is that vibrations produced at the eardrum by electrical methods are perceived in the inner ear in the same way as acoustical vibration.'

Rutschmann [10] and Rutschmann et al. [11] studied electromagnetic stimulation of the eardrum by gluing a 10-mg magnet (Cunico) on the umbo of normal hearing subjects. The magnet was driven by an electromagnetic field produced by an oscillator and externally worn coil. The coil was 7 cm in internal diameter and was worn on the pinna 3–4 cm from the magnet. The air-conduction threshold at 1,000 Hz was 0 dB HL (RE ISO 1964) while the corresponding induction threshold was 7.9 mA of coil current. Radio programs were monitored using the induction system and the subject claimed 'reproduction was satisfactory'.

Glorig et al. [12] glued a magnet on the umbo in one subject and using an external amplifier and coil found that speech was heard 'with a clarity comparable to sounds heard when wearing earphones'.

The principle of the electromagnetic implant hearing aid is shown in figure 1. Sounds enter the microphone of amplifier A and are transformed into an electromagnetic field produced by coil B. The field acts to move magnet C, which is attached to the malleus, incus or stapes so that sound is produced.

We have previously published results using electromagnetic induction hearing in 8 human subjects [4–7]. In 1970 [4] we studied 1 normal subject with exceptional hearing using a small stimulating coil deep in the ear canal, 3 mm from a 50-mg Alnico V magnet glued on the umbo. The coil had a resistance of 580 Ω and an inductance of 65 mH and was connected to a pure tone generator. In this subject –10 dB HL equivalent thresholds at 500, 1,000 and 2,000 Hz were reached with 0.7 μA mean peak-to-peak coil current. Until recently we have been unable to duplicate this efficiency and suspect his actual hearing threshold was –20 dB HL or better.

In 1973 [5] we evaluated 3 normal hearing subjects with different weight (10–55 mg) Alnico V magnets glued on the umbo. The magnet was energized by an air-cored 2.4 cm outer diameter coil located about 3 cm from the magnet on the postauricular skin. The coil consisted of 150 turns of No. 32 copper wire with a resistance of 6 Ω. The mean peak-to-peak induction current threshold for the group was 0.62 mA at 500, 1,000 and 2,000 Hz and 0.68 mA for the SRT. The mean hearing threshold for the group at 500, 1,000 and 2,000 Hz was 10 dB HL. Speech discrimination scores obtained using a microphone and speech amplifier attached to the coil were equivalent to scores obtained using live voice air-conduction speech testing with W-22 word lists under earphones. The 55-mg magnet gave the best results.

A fourth subject was studied in the operating room during tympanotomy for tympanic nerve section. A sterile 55-mg Alnico V magnet was placed in turn on the umbo, long process of the incus, and round window membrane. Induction pure tone thresholds at the standard audiometric frequencies were obtained for each site using a postauricular coil connected to the pure tone generator. Placement of the sterile magnet on the long process of the incus and round window membrane after tympanotomy produced the same induction thresholds as the umbo site. There appeared to be no site advantage in this subject.

A fifth subject with a mild sensorineural loss had a more permanent type of magnet placement. A Silverstein malleus-clip prosthesis was used to house a 85-mg Alnico V magnet and attached in the usual manner to the malleus handle. This apparatus was in place for 22 months without incident and evaluations of its effectiveness were performed regularly

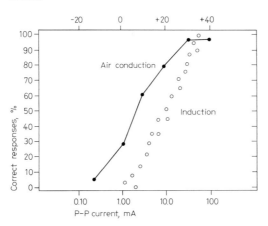

Fig.2. Air conduction stimulus intensity, dB re: SRT.

over a 12-month period. The hearing thresholds at 500, 1,000 and 2,000 Hz were 15, 30 and 55 dB HL while the induction thresholds at 500, 1,000 and 2,000 Hz were 2.3, 2.0 and 5.1 mA peak-to-peak current in the coil. Thresholds could not be obtained at 4,000 Hz with either method. This subject could use a body-worn hearing aid connected to the coil behind the ear capable of providing 100 mA output.

Figure 2 gives his performance-intensity function for air conduction and electromagnetic induction delivered PB words. It shows that both systems were equivalent (>96%); the SRT threshold ranged from 1 to 3 mA during the test period. Loading of the tympanic membrane with a 55-mg magnet or the 85-mg Silverstein tube and magnet combination did not produce any change in air-conduction thresholds up to and including 4,000 Hz. Higher frequencies may be adversely affected by increased mass so we prefer the magnet to weigh 50 mg or less.

The postauricular coil location was chosen in these subjects because it left the ear canal completely open and cosmetically oppeared to be an improvement. It was dramatically less efficient than the intracanal location.

In 1978 [6] we evaluated another normal hearing subject using a system similar to that studied in 1970, but with a 50-mg platinum cobalt magnet on the umbo. 0.02 mA peak-to-peak coil current was required to achieve an equivalent hearing threshold of 5 dB HL at 1,000 Hz. Speech discrimination for live voice, 50 word, W-22 word lists presented under earphones and via the induction system were again equivalent (100 vs. 96%).

In 1986 [7], using a 50-mg samarium cobalt magnet on the umbo with a substantially higher magnetic energy product than platinum cobalt or Alnico and improved coil design, we achieved thresholds equivalent to 80 dB HL at 1,000 Hz with 3,5 mA RMS in the coil. The coil location in the canal was the same as in the 1970 and 1978 experiments [4, 6]. This system could be used in mild hearing loss patients with a behind the ear aid.

Since energy transfer between the coil and magnet falls off inversely with the cube of the distance [13], location of the coil deep in the ear canal seems optimal. For maximum efficiency, the coil should lie as close as possible to the magnet, ideally, surrounding it. The coil should be oriented so that the magnet points toward the center of the coil. The coil should not occlude the ear canal nor produce pain or trauma to the canal or tympanic membrane. The magnet should be as strong as possible. Whereas in our long-term subject the magnet was attached to the umbo, it might be better for the magnet to be implanted in the middle ear cavity in contact with the malleus, incus or stapes. This would eliminate any problems with water, ear wax or desquamated skin in the ear canal producing irritation or infection around the magnet.

Additional testing the past two years using a canal coil of improved design and more powerful rare earth magnets suggests that the inefficiency between coil and magnet can be further improved so that an in the ear device can be developed with a reasonable power requirement and battery life. The status of the efficiency of the published coil-magnet systems is shown in table I. The reason that a practical electromagnetic induction air conduction hearing aid does not exist to date has been because of the inefficiency of the coupling between coil and magnet. This appears to be solved at least for mild to moderate losses.

One difficulty with an electromagnetic induction hearing system is that the inductive reactance of the coil increases directly with frequency so that with each doubling of frequency, a 6-dB decrease in current through the coil occurs for the same voltage input. This must be offset by increased output from the amplifier at higher frequencies.

The question of improved speech fidelity with a partially implanted aid needs more study. The best data regarding the relative speech fidelity of a system that directly drives the ossicles versus a conventional amplifying system were obtained in guinea pigs by Mahoney and Vernon [14]. In

Table I. Status of the efficiency of various coil-magnet systems

Year of study	Reference	Coil current in mA (RMS) to produce 80 dB HL at 1,000 Hz	Magnet material	Coil location
1959	10	28,000	Cunico	pinna
1970	4	7,8	Alnico V	ear canal
1973	5	2,200	Alnico V	post-auricular
1978	6	40	platinum cobalt	ear canal
1986	7	3,5	samarium cobalt	ear canal

experiments using animals with noise-induced high frequency hair cell damage, they found that speech materials presented by driving the incus directly with a piezoelectric rod produced discrimination scores 18% better than when the same materials were presented with conventional audiometry. The responses were compared by recording the round window cochlear microphonic produced by the speech stimuli in both conditions and using them as test materials for normal listeners. We have reported results in 5 subjects where a subjective comparison was made [5]. All of the subjects preferred induction-produced speech to audiometer-produced speech. No significant differences in speech discrimination were found between the two methods; however, testing was done only in quiet [5]. This has also been our experience in more recent testing; when properly performed, induction hearing is preferred.

The use of this induction system for the correction of conductive losses needs some discussion. The magnet can be incorporated in a variety of incus and incus-stapes replacement prostheses used to reconstruct the middle ear. We feel that partially implantable aids designed to correct conductive hearing losses have promise at this time. The encapsulated magnet can be inserted at the time of tympanomastoid or middle ear surgery if it appears that ossicular reconstruction is not likely to restore thesholds to 30 dB HL or better in the speech frequency range of 500–4,000 Hz. If a satisfactory hearing level is not achieved following surgery, the electromagnetic induction hearing aid could be used to drive the magnet in the prosthesis, correcting any residual conductive loss.

Frederickson et al. [15] and Hough et al. [16, 17] have described a more complex scheme of electromagnetic induction hearing where the stimulating coil is implanted in the middle ear or mastoid cavity very close to the magnet attached to an ossicle. This coil is connected to a second, larger coil implanted under the postauricular skin. A third primary coil is on the skin surface just over this second coil and connected to the external hearing aid. The implant coils are energized by electromagnetic induction or radio frequency transmission via the primary coil. This is similar to the system described by Yanagihara et al. [18] to energize a piezoelectric implant. In this version, there is a loss of energy at two locations instead of one.

Electromagnetic Bone Conduction Hearing Aids

A partially implantable bone conduction (BC) hearing aid has been developed in which an encapsulated samarium cobalt magnet attached to a bone screw is screwed into the cortex of the mastoid bone under the postauricular skin [17]. After healing, an external coil attached to a body-worn hearing aid is placed over the implant magnet and held in place by a small magnet in the center of the external coil. Speech is amplified by the aid and converted to an electromagnetic field by the coil, producing vibration of the implant magnet and skull. Subjects with a conductive hearing loss whose BC thresholds are 25 dB HL or better can benefit from the device. The large size of the external aid is a disadvantage but an on-the-ear version is expected by late 1987. Another bone conduction aid developed in Sweden uses a small osseo-integrated titanium screw passing through the skin over the mastoid bone into the mastoid cortex [19]. A behind-the-ear hearing aid with vibrator output connects to an attachment on the screw. Patients with a conductive hearing loss and BC thresholds better than 40 dB HL can benefit from the device. The fidelity and convenience may be better than conventional bone conduction hearing aids and certainly have promise in cases of congenital atresia and inoperable conductive losses.

Conventional bone conduction hearing aids have not been well accepted in the United States for conductive hearing loss due to difficulty in maintaining proper pressure between the bone conduction transducer and mastoid without a head spring; the spring, while effective, is cosmetically unattractive. Eyeglass bone conduction aids offer a solution, if eyeglasses are normally worn all the time, but have difficulty maintaining the proper pressure on the mastoid. On or in-the-ear air conduction aids are more commonly prescribed for conductive or mixed losses for this reason but because they occlude the ear canal they can contribute to recurrent otitis externa and produce drainage in patients who have had prior tympanomastoid surgery for chronic otitis media. As mentioned previously, the use of partially implantable bone conduction aids in children with bilateral atretic ears is a potential indication since reconstruction of these cases often fails to achieve normal hearing thresholds in the 500–4,000 Hz range. In theory, a super-efficient bone conduction aid, such as the Swedish transcutaneous version mounted on a bone screw in the mastoid cortex [19], could be used for mild sensorineural hearing losses without a conductive component. Testing to date has not shown this to be the case; thresholds cannot be improved significantly above the bone conduction level.

Additional work is required to verify whether a partially implantable aid that directly drives the ossicles is superior to a conventional hearing aid and, if so, by how much and under what circumstances. Whereas many of the subjects who have used these experimental devices comment on the excellent sound clarity compared with conventional aids, further data are needed.

References

1   Miller, J. D.; Niemoeller, A. F.: Hearing aid design and evaluation for a patient with a severe discrimination loss for speech. J. Speech Hear. Res. *10:* 367–372 (1967).

2   Dodds, E., Hartford, E.: Modified earpieces and CROS for high frequency hearing losses. J. Speech Hear. Res. *2 204–218* (1968)

3   Schuneman, J. R.: Viscomi, G. J.: Open canal amplification. Trans. Am. Acad. Ophtal. Otolar. *78:* 256–260 (1974).

4   Goode, R. L.: An implantable hearing aid: state of the art. Trans. Am. Acad. Ophtal. Otolar. *74:* 128–139 (1970).

5   Goode, R. L.; Glattke, T.: Audition via electromagnetic induction. Archs Otolar. *98:* 23–26 (1973).

6   Goode, R. L.: Implantable hearing aids. Otolaryngol. Clin. North Am. *11:* 155–161 (1978).

7   Goode, R. L.; Aritomo, H.; Gonzales, J.; Gyo, K.: The implantable hearing aid; in Van Steenberghe, Tissue integration in oral maxillo-facial reconstruction, pp. 199–208 (Excerpta Medica, Amsterdam 1986).

8   Wilska, A.: Eine Methode zur Bestimmung der Hörschwellenamplituden des Trommelfells bei verschiedenen Frequenzen. Skand. Arch. Physiol. 72: 161–165 (1935).
9   Wilska, A.: A direct method for determining threshold amplitudes of the eardrum at various frequencies; in Kobrak, The middle ear, pp. 76–79 (University of Chicago Press, Chicago 1959).
10   Rutschmann, J.: Magnetic audition-auditory stimulation by means of alternating magnetic fields acting on a permanent magnet fixed to the eardrum. IRE Trans Med. Electronics 6: 22–23 (1959).
11   Rutschmann, J.; Page, H. J.; Fowler, E. P. jr.: Auditory stimulation: alternating magnetic fields acting on a permanent magnet fixed to the eardrum. Read before the American Physiological Society Meeting, Philadelphia 1958.
12   Glorig, A., et al.: Magnetically coupled stimulation of the ossicular chain: measures in kangaroo rat and man. J. Acoust. Soc. Am. 52: 694–696 (1972).
13   Mackay, R. S.: Bio-medical telemetry, pp. 1–351 (Wiley, New York 1986).
14   Mahoney, T.; Vernon, J.: Speech induced cochlear potentials. Archs Otolar. 100: 403–404 (1974).
15   Frederickson, J. M., et al: Evaluation of an electromagnetic implantable hearing aid. Can. J. Otolaryngol. 2: (1973).
16   Hough, J.; Vernon, J.; Meikel, M.; Himelick, T.; Richard, G.; Dormer, K.: A middle ear implantable hearing device for controlled amplification of sound in the human: a preliminary report. Laryngoscope 97: 141–151 (1987).
17   Hough, J.; Vernon, J.; Dormer, K.; Johnson, B.; Himelick, T.: Experiences with implantable hearing devices and a presentation of a new device. Ann. Otol. Rhinol. Lar. 1: 60–65 (1986).
18   Yanagihara, H.; Suzuki, J.; Gyo, K.; Syono, H.; Ikeda, H.: Development of an implantable hearing aid using a piezoelectric vibrator of bimorph design: state of the art. Otolar. Head Neck Surg. 92: 706 (1984).
19   Hakansson, B.; Tjellström, A.; Rosenhall, U.: Hearing thresholds with direct bone conduction versus conventional bone conduction. Scand. Audiol. 13: 3–13 (1984).

Richard L. Goode, MD, Division of Otolaryngology, Department of Surgery, Stanford University Medical Center, Stanford, CA 94305 (USA)

Adv. Audiol., vol. 4, pp. 32–43 (Karger, Basel 1988)

Development of a Semi-Implantable Hearing Device

Jorgen Heide, Gary Tatge, Tom Sander, Tim Gooch, Tony Prescott

Richards Medical Company, Memphis, Tenn., USA

Introduction

Hearing-impaired persons number approximately five hundred million worldwide. Only an estimated four million hearing aids are sold annually on the world market. Many of the remaining hearing-impaired individuals are potentially good candidates for hearing assistance but resist seeking medical/audiological help because, for many, traditional hearing aids are cosmetically unacceptable. Unfortunately, most current hearing aid designs fall into this category because they carry the stigma of aging, physical handicap or the false assumption that there is an inability of the user to perform many day-to-day functions as well as a normal-hearing person. Also, there are a number of performance issues that make current hearing aid technology unacceptable – limited frequency response, unwanted distortion and acoustic feedback, just to name a few.

Conventional hearing aids function by converting sound into electrical signals, processing and amplifying these signals before they are converted back into amplified acoustic sound. Energy lost due to friction and damping in the transducers causes the amplified sound to have a poorer quality than the original sound, even though it is louder. By reducing these losses and other side effects in the output transducer, the amplified sound would have a better quality.

Despite great strides in conventional hearing aid technology, several research studies have demonstrated that implantable hearing devices using non acoustic transducers may provide many hearing-impaired individuals with superior results than would be obtainable with conventional acoustic transducers. Goode [1] and Goode and Glattke [2] conducted studies using an electromagnetic induction system and reported greatly reduced distortion levels, which many be linked to improved speech discrimination, better sound quality, reduction of acoustic feedback and a vast reduction in patient concern for the cosmetic acceptance of the assistive device. Frederickson et al. [3] also conducted experiments on electromagnetic hearing devices in the early 1970s. The major obstacles faced by these researchers were miniaturization of the electrical components and the electromagnetic power available to drive implanted magnets. Yanagihara et al. [4, 5] have developed a piezoelectric device which can directly stimulate the ossicular chain. More recently, Hough et al. [6, 7] have developed a bone-conduction hearing aid which relies on a magnet implanted into the skull to enhance sound vibrations traveling to the cochlea.

With these considerations in mind, Richards Medical Company initiated a major project to develop an electromagnetic hearing device which would be, for all practical purposes, minimally invasive and totally invisible from outside the body. Laboratory and clinical testing revealed solutions to problems that may have prevented others from achieving a realistic device.

Device Description

This device consists of two major components: an electronic battery-operated driver unit and a small implantable rare-earth magnet.

The electronic driver system and electromagnetic output transducer (coil) are encased in a custom housing produced from an impression of the patient's ear. This is similar to the process frequently used to produce housings for small conventional custom canal hearing aids. A negative cast is made from the same impression duplicating the patient's external ear canal. This cast is later used as a jig to permanently fix the distance from the tip of the driver unit to the patient's tympanic membrane, as well as align the output transducer with the permanent magnet.

The custom housing which fits inconspicuously into the patient's ear canal contains all the components required in the driver system. A small electret microphone is used to convert incoming sound energy into electrical signals. These signals are then amplified, processed, compressed and frequency spectrum-shaped before entering an output stage where a conversion into analog magnetic signals takes place. This is what then drives the electromagnetic transducer. These magnetic signals are finally directed toward the implanted magnet. The entire driver system is powered by a small, single-cell, conventional canal hearing aid battery.

Designing the driver unit to fit into the external canal allows the patient to easily remove the unit for battery replacement, as well as eliminating amplification at night should they desire not to hear while asleep. This type of design also eliminates many of the potential problems raised in earlier studies such as battery replacement, access to the electronics for possible service, repairs, technology upgrades and placement of the electret microphone. The tip of the custom housing is tapered to eliminate any discomfort from physical contact with the sensitive, bony portion of the external auditory canal.

The second major component is an implantable rare-earth samarium-cobalt (Sm-Co) magnet. This material is an alloy of $SmCo_5$ which has been used extensively as an implantable magnetic material in the past and has shown to be essentially nontoxic in biocompatibility studies. As an additional precaution and to ensure long-term corrosion resistance, the magnet is coated with materials already being used extensively to isolate other implantable devices from body fluids. The magnet is shaped as a small disc with a diameter of 2.5–3.0 mm and a total weight between 25 and 35 mg.

The analog magnetic signals produced by the output transducer are directed toward the implantable magnet causing it to vibrate in correspondence with the amplified sound. This amplified motion applied to the middle ear creates the audible sound effect to the patient similar to the sound effect generated by movements of the tympanic membrane by acoustic force. Since the sound effect generated by the semi-implantable hearing device does not use acoustic energy, potential feedback is eliminated. This will allow maximum venting of the device for pressure equalization and patient comfort. Irregularities in the frequency response of most acoustic output transducers are also eliminated, improving the sound reproduction quality over conventional hearing aids.

In vitro Testing

Over the years, standardized audiological test procedures have been established using acoustic stimuli referenced to known sound pressure levels. Similarly, performance characteristics of conventional hearing aids are reported with reference to sound pressure levels, using various standards such as ANSI in the United States and IEC methods throughout the world.

Since no acoustic energy is present at the output of the semi-implantable hearing device driver unit, extensive laboratory work was performed to convert magnetic force and movement of the magnet into equivalent sound pressure levels in order to establish performance data and fitting guidelines for the device.

Measurements of equivalent sound pressure levels were conducted by attaching the permanent magnet to a piezoelectric ceramic transducer and directly correlating the electrical signals from that transducer to a reference acoustic measuring microphone (Bruel & Kjaer 2642). Using a CF-920 FFT Analyzer, various measuring microphone amplifiers and mathematical computations to adjust for any nonlinear characteristics which may have occurred due to the inertial effects of the mass of the magnet, these data were directly converted to sound pressure levels.

The performance of the device is naturally related to the distance between the output driver and the magnet. In vivo testing has shown that this distance can be established and adjusted according to the power requirements while maintaining a safe distance between the driver and tympanic membrane, approximately 2.5–5.0 mm.

Performing the in vitro testing just described and using ANSI S3.22–1982 guidelines, the following data were obtained.

These data indicate a possible fitting range of sensorineural hearing loss from mild to moderately severe.

SSPL 90 (maximum output)	100–115 dB SPL
High-frequency average SSPL 90	95–110 dB SPL
Full-on gain	30–50 dB
High frequency average full-on gain	35–45 dB
Reference test gain	23–38 dB
Frequency range	150–10,000 Hz
Total harmonic distortion	<2%
Battery current	1.3 V, 900 μA (0.9 mA)

SSPL 90 = saturated sound pressure using 90 dB SPL of input; SPL = sound pressure level.

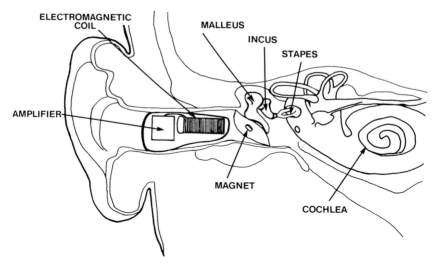

Fig. 1. Richards semi-implantable hearing device in situ in external acoustic meatus. For testing purposes the Sm-Co magnet was glued to the tympanic membrane with New Skin.

In vivo Testing

Human trials were conducted to answer the following questions.

(1) Is nonacoustic energy efficiently coupled to the middle ear system with sufficient gain and output characteristics necessary to fit a typical sensorineural hearing loss?

(2) Is there a perceived improvement of the sound quality versus conventional hearing aid systems?

(3) Is there a significant reduction or elimination in acoustic feedback?

In order to answer these questions, two Investigational Review Board (IRB) approvals were obtained from two independent medical institutions. The IRB study proposal outlined a procedure of minimal risk to the patients and allowed for accurate, clinical data collection which would have been impossible to obtain through any animal or laboratory study. Six patients participated in the study (three from each institution), all of who exhibited 'typical' sensorineural hearing loss configurations bilaterally. One patient (B. G.) had normal hearing through 2,000 Hz, with only a 4,000 Hz high-frequency component to his hearing loss. Objective and subjective patient data were collected and compared to both unaided and aided responses. These data will be reported and discussed later in this paper.

The study employed patients who were hearing aid users with sensorineural hearing loss of no more than 70 dB. Each patient was tested for sensitivity to an adhesive New Skin® by placing a small drop to the forearm 2–3 weeks before placement of the magnet. The skin patch test results were reviewed by the attending physician prior to being accepted for this study. Next, a deep ear mold impression was taken and sent to Richards Medical Company to assist in the manufacture of the custom-fit driver system.

Coated Sm-Co magnets ranging in weight from 35 to 46.4 mg were attached using New Skin as an adhesive to the lateral surface of the tympanic membrane at the umbo. After the magnet was in place and the New Skin allowed to dry, each patient was thoroughly tested using standard audiometric techniques. After full audiometric evaluations, each patient was allowed to wear the unit for a period of time and in a variety of listening environments to determine his or her subjective experience to the amplified sound. Results of the audiometric testing and subjective evaluations will be discussed in this report. Figure 1 shows the system in place in the ear.

Audiometric test procedures consisted of sound field warbled-tone audiograms performed pre- and post-magnet attachment to determine if there was any loading effect or impedance changes that resulted in sensitivity losses due to the mass of the magnet on the tympanic membrane. Electroacoustic impedance test studies were also performed pre- and post-magnet attachment to confirm or reject this possibility. Sound field threshholds were taken with the implanted unit and compared to threshholds with the patients' existing hearing aid. Speech discrimination was measured using the electromagnetic implant and compared to aided and unaided performance.

Clinical Results

For the purposes of this study, pure tone comparisons were made between baseline audiograms, the implant and the patients' current hearing aid. As can be observed in table I, the implant does produce significant amounts of functional gain for all 6 patients. At only one frequency

Table I. Functional gain analysis (dB)

Patients	Frequency, kHz				
	0.25	0.5	1.0	2.0	4.0
F.S.					
Hearing aid	0	−5	5	15	20
Implant	10	20	25	20	−10
W.A.					
Hearing aid	0	0	5	15	15
Implant	15	30	25	30	15
G.D.					
Hearing aid	0	0	15	25	15
Implant	20	30	35	35	25
C.M.					
Hearing aid	0	5	25	30	10
Implant	35	45	40	35	−25
P.S.					
Hearing aid	5	−10	5	15	30
Implant	35	30	25	25	20
B.G.					
Hearing aid	0	5	0	0	15
Implant	15	10	0	5	10
Average gain					
Hearing aid	0.83	−0.83	9.17	16.67	17.50
Implant	21.66	27.50	25.00	25.00	5.83
Difference	20.83	28.33	15.83	8.33	−11.67

(4,000 Hz) did the patients' existing hearing aid produce more functional gain, on the average, than the electromagnet implant device. This result was skewed somewhat by patient C.M. who was the only patient who scored significantly lower than his baseline threshhold with the implant and this was only observed at one frequency, 4,000 Hz.

In the important speech frequencies of 500, 1,000 and 2,000 Hz, the implant produced an average of 17.5 dB of functional gain improvement over their current hearing aid. This fact can also be demonstrated in the speech reception threshhold testing (table II) in which an average improvement of 10.8 dB of speech sensitivity improvement was obtained us-

Table II. Speech evaluation analysis: Improvement (dB) in speech reception threshold

Patient	Hearing aid	Implant	Difference
F.S.	5	20	15
W.A.	0	10	10
G.D.	15	30	15
C.M.	25	35	10
P.S.	12	27	15
B.G.	5	5	0
Average improvement (dB) 10.33		21.17	10.84

Table III. Speech discrimination: Improvement from unaided score

Patient	Improvement, %		
	hearing aid	implant	difference
F.S.	16	16	0
W.A.	24	52	28
G.D.	80	80	0
C.M.	0	–4	–4
P.S.	36	32	–4
B.G.	8	4	–4
Average improvement	27.53	30.00	2.67

ing the implant. There were no patients in the study that exhibited poorer speech reception threshholds with the implant versus the hearing aid.

Speech discrimination was also measured (table III). One patient scored significantly better with his implant than with his hearing aid (28%). With the other 5 patients, no significant differences were found between hearing aid performance and the electromagnetic implant. On the average, however, there was a 30% improvement over their baseline unaided speech discrimination scores using the electromagnetic implant.

An analysis of each patients' subjective postimplant questionnaires revealed several common characteristics of the implant. First, the implant appears to have a different type of sound than traditional hearing aids. The patients report a very quiet, more natural type of sound. Second, most patients reported difficulty with their hearing aids in noisy environments. Based on the subjective responses, it appears that the implant performs extremely well in a wide variety of noisy situations. Third, none of the patients experienced problems with acoustic feedback during their evaluation process.

During the evaluation, attempts were made to increase the functional gain delivered by the patients' conventional hearing aid to more closely match that of the semi-implantable hearing device. In each case, we discovered that one or more of the following occurred: (1) adding more gain typically produced feedback; (2) the patients were generally displeased by the increased loudness of the aid even with additional venting, low-frequency roll-off and optimized compression, and (3) at the increased gain settings, the standard hearing aids were not able to process noisy environments as well as the magnetic device.

The quantitative differences between the baseline audiograms, the implant and the hearing aid responses are apparent in the pure tone testing. Qualitative differences, on the other hand, are somewhat more difficult to measure, but there appears to be some commonality in the subjective responses of the patients. The difference in sound quality may be due to the type of transducers, the electromagnetic coupling of sound to the middle ear system, the lower distortion characteristics or a combination of these factors. Future research in electromagnetic amplification may help identify answers to why the patients' subjective experiences were so good.

Permanent Implantable Devices

Two versions of this hearing device are presently being constructed, one for conductive or mixed losses where ossicular replacement surgery is recommended regardless of the availability of this device and a second version for sensorineural hearing losses. The difference between the two versions are the implantable parts of the device while the driver unit remains identical.

The first version was developed using the information gained from the previously described studies. The 'electromagnetic ossicular replacement device' is designed for patients who are candidates for partial ossicular replacement prosthesis or total ossicular replacement prosthesis (TORP). Figure 2 shows the magnetic TORP which is similar to currently

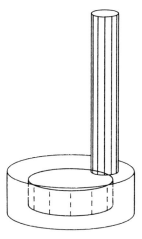

Fig. 2. Magnetic TORP, similar to currently marketed TORPs, with a modified base plate to accommodate the magnet.

marketed Richards TORPs with a modification to accommodate the magnet. Figure 3 shows this device placed in a patient's ear.

The second version is being designed to be implanted into a healthy middle ear, preserve the ossicles and provide amplification for purely sensorineural hearing losses. Figure 4 shows the device for sensorineural hearing losses using a specially-constructed magnet system which can be placed on the long process of the incus in the middle ear.

It is expected these two permanent implant versions will perform at least equal to and possibly somewhat better than indicated by the study conducted with the magnet temporarily glued on the tympanic membrane. This is based on a theory that part of the motion of the small magnet placed on a large flexible tympanic membrane is absorbed by the system while the rigid attachment, in the two final versions of this product, will transfer more of the motion energy to the oval window of the chochlea. Some minor changes to the driver unit should further increase high-frequency performance.

Conclusion

Technological advances in hearing aid design over the past several years have primarily focused attention on automatic signal processing

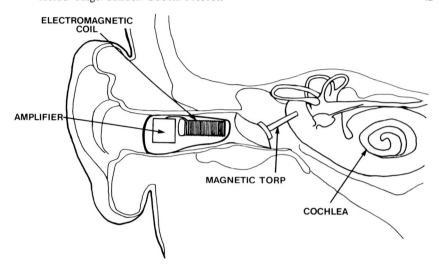

Fig. 3. Richards semi-implantable hearing device in combination with magnetic TORP in situ.

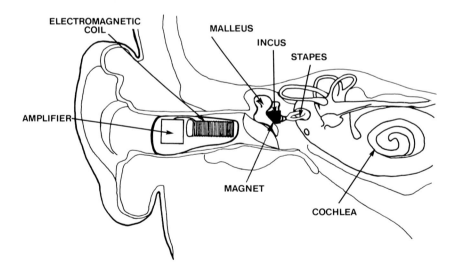

Fig. 4. Richards semi-implantable hearing device adapted to sensorineural hearing losses using a magnet system placed on the long process of the incus.

and electronic circuit miniaturization. These advances have brought about smaller, more sophisticated hearing aid designs, but have left many problems unsolved. For example, the common yet unwanted by-product of the miniaturization of hearing aids has been the problem of acoustic feedback. Efforts to produce the ideal cosmetic package for a hearing aid are continually restricted by this problem. A second major concern is that acoustic transducers may be responsible for much of the distortional characteristics present in traditional hearing aids. Exchanging the acoustic output transducer for a lower-distortion device may improve the overall sound quality and ultimately the patient's acceptance of the device.

Based on our experiences developing and testing the present electromagnetic semi-implantable hearing device, both primary problems of feedback and distortion can be minimized or eliminated. This, in conjunction with a highly cosmetic package, can present the hearing-impaired community with a viable alternative to traditional acoustic hearing aids. Many of our early clinical successes with the current semi-implantable hearing device have provided us with great optimism for the very near future.

References

1 Goode, R. L.: An implantable hearing aid – state of the art. Trans Am. Acad. Ophthal. Otolar. *74:* 128–139 (1970).
2 Goode, R. L.; Glattke, T. J.: Audition via electromagnetic induction. Archs Otolar. *98:* 23–26 (1973).
3 Fredrickson, J. M.; Tomlinson, D. R.; Davis, E. R.; Odkirst, L. M.: Evaluation of an electromagnetic implantable hearing aid. Can. J. Otolaryngol. *2:* 53–62 (1973).
4 Yanagihara, N.; Suzuki, K.; Gyo, K.; Araki, H.: Perception of sound through direction oscillation of the stapes using a piezoelectric ceramic bimorph. Ann. Otol. Rhinol. Lar. *92:* 223–227 (1983).
5 Yanagihara, N.; et al.: Development of an implantable hearing aid using a piezoelectric vibrator of bimorph design: state of the art. Otolar. Head Neck Surg. *92:* 706–712 (1984).
6 Hough, J.; Himelick, T.; Johnson, B.: Implantable bone conduction hearing device: audiant bone conductor – update on our experiences. Ann. Otol. Rhinol. Lar. *95:* 498–504 (1986).
7 Hough, J.; Vernon, J.; Johnson, B.; Dormer, K.; Himelick, T.: Experiences with implantable hearing devices and a presentation of a new device. Ann. Otol. Rhinol. Lar. *95:* 60–65 (1986).

Jorgen Heide, Richards Medical Company, Memphis, TN (USA)

Adv. Audiol., vol. 4, pp. 44–50 (Karger, Basel 1988)

Vibratory Stimulation of the Cochlea through a Percutaneous Transducer

Anders Tjellström

Department of Otolaryngology, Sahlgren's Hospital,
University of Göteborg, Sweden

The totally implanted hearing aid has for many years been a challenge for the otologist. During the last decade problems related to reach this goal have been approached from different angles. A great body of knowledge and experience from animal research as well as clinical trials has been collected and the international discussions in this field have increased every year. The idea to publish the present state of art in *Advances in Audiology* is an indication of this growing interest.

To be asked by Prof. Suzuki to present our view on this matter is a great honour and pleasure. It should be made clear that the results that we have achieved are a good example of interdisciplinary cooperation, a necessity to reach results in this field. The institutions that have significantly contributed to the results in this presentation are: the Ear-Nose-Throat (ENT) Department of Sahlgren's Hospital. University of Göteborg; the Institute for Applied Biotechnology, Göteborg; the Department of Applied Electronics, Chalmers University of Technology, Göteborg, and Nobelpharma Company, Göteborg, Sweden.

Discussions with several scientists from different fields have taken place over the years and have likewise been of utmost importance in the development of our contribution, a transducer connected to an osseo-integrated titanium implant through a percutaneous coupling.

The majority of papers in this volume are focused on a direct stimulation of a mobile stapes footplate with or without superstructures. The only device which has been tested so far is the partial middle ear implant. The energy source for this implant is through induction coils. The external device includes two coils, microphone, electronics and a battery. No reports of clinical tests with the total middle ear implant have been published as of June, 1987.

Some problems related to total middle ear implants could be identified.

(1) Microphone. Where is the optimal placement of the microphone? What type of soft tissue should cover it? What degree of fidelity can be reached with such a placement?

(2) Switches/controls. How will the on/off switch be placed? It is well-known that patients using hearing aids frequently change the volume depending on the listening situation. Some possibilities for the patient to adjust the TMei might be necessary.

(3) Energy source. An implanted battery with connector is needed that are both safe and corrosion-resistant. Should it be rechargeable through the skin?

All these problems could very easily be solved if a lasting skin penetration could be established.

Since 1977, at the ENT Department of Sahlgren's Hospital, Göteborg, we have been using titanium implants with percutaneous connectors for attaching bone-conduction hearing aids as well as retention of craniofacial prostheses. Several papers have been published over the years discussing osseointegration from various aspects and with detailed descriptions of the procedures and the results [1–12]. In this chapter only data relevant to the middle ear implants will be discussed.

Osseointegration

In order to establish and permanently maintain a reaction-free skin penetration it is necessary to reduce the movements of the skin in relation to the implant. This could best be achieved through an implant secured to the bone tissue and thin skin adherent to the surrounding bone. Osseointegration has been defined by Brånemark [10] as 'a direct structural-functional connection between ordered living bone and the surface of a load-carrying implant'. To establish this direct contact between organized Haversian bone and an implant several factors have to be taken into consideration.

The *implant material* is of great importance, of course. Based on theoretical aspects as well as clinical experience, commercially pure titanium has been used in our work. When titanium is processed the surface is coated with an oxide layer which is responsible for the chemistry at the implant/biotissue interface. The chemical inertness and the high dielectric constant of titanium oxide are important factors contributing to the high biocompatibility of titanium implants [9]. The oxide film is also very dense and its attachment to the bulk metal very good.

The *implant design* is another factor of importance. We are using a screw-shaped implant that will provide a good and very important stability during the initial healing period and also will result in a larger surface area.

The *surgical technique* has been designed in a way to minimize the surgical trauma to the implant bed. If this trauma is not kept under control a fibrous capsule might be formed between the implant and the Haversian bone. Such a fibrous attachment could function at the beginning, but as time goes by and a especially if a load is put on the implant the risk of implant loss is very high.

Other factors of importance are the *microstructure* of the implant surface, *status of the implant bed* and the *loading conditions*. All these factors have been discussed in detail by Albrektsson et al. [5].

Skin Penetration

In order to establish and permanently maintain a reaction-free skin penetration two prerequisites are of special importance.

First, the skin round the implant should not move in relation to the implant. To achieve this an extensive subcutaneous tissue reduction is performed and the very thin skin should adhere to the bone surface. The ideal situation to imitate is a thin graft covering a bony surface after tumor surgery.

Second, the skin-penetrating area should be free of hair follicles. This could be achieved with a rotation flap or a free skin graft taken from the fold behind the ear or from the inside of the upper arm.

Clinical Experience

The experience with percutaneous implants in clinical practice goes back to 1977. Since then, more than 400 implants penetrating the skin have been placed in the mastoid process. More than 150 of these have been followed for a longer period than 4 years. The reasons for this type of implant surgery have been for retention of auricular prostheses and for attaching bone-conduction hearing aids directly to the bone. An analysis of the status of the skin around these implants has been performed and published [12]. Of a total of 708 observations, 61 had some sign of adverse skin reaction, which corresponds to 8.6%. If only significant adverse reaction is calculated there were only 34 of 708 observations (4.8%). Failure rate calculated over time is generally done when discussing longevity of cardiac pacemakers. For cardiac pacemakers the failure rate is often in the range of 0.02–0.04% per month. Holgers et al. [12] found in their study a failure rate for percutaneous implants of 0.14% per month. Our conclusion is that using the right implant material with an appropriate design and a surgical technique adjusted to the very special demands it is possible to establish and maintain a reaction-free skin penetration in most patients.

Vibratory Tests on the Otic Capsule

In an ongoing study we are measuring the hearing threshold for pure tones (500–8,000 Hz) in patients for different positions of a transducer in the temporal bone. Preliminary results indicate that the closer the vibrator is to the otic capsule the lesser is the energy needed to reach the threshold.

The gain has been found to be more than 10 times when the transducer is placed on the otic capsule as compared to when the mastoid cortex is stimulated [Tjellström et al., in preparation]. Some of the tested patients also indicate a better fidelity of the sound as the transducer approaches the cochlea. Of course, this is still bone conduction and with a transducer direct on the stapes foot-plate a much greater gain could be anticipated. Working on the foot-plate could, however, be hazardous as it always includes a risk, even if it is small, for a permanent cochlear damage.

Future Considerations

Two different possibilities to combine the experiences discussed above could be identified. The first is to use the principle of vibrating the stapes with a piezoelectric bimorph as developed by Suzuki et al. [13] and Yanagihara et al. [14]. This device could very easily be combined with an

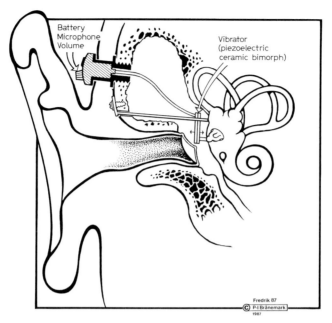

Fig. 1. Schematic drawing of a piezoelectric bimorph inducing vibrations to the stapes. The energy is provided through a percutaneous connector attached to an osseo-integrated titanium implant.

titanium implant integrated in the bone and equipped with a percutaneous coupling. Such an arrangement would eliminate the space-occupying internal coils as well as insulation and package problems. The risk of leakage from a subcutaneously placed unit would also be eliminated. As illustrated in figure 1, the battery, microphone and the volume controls could be placed in one unit easy to reach by the patient. The electronics could possibly also be placed in this coupling without any difficulties, and a significant problem related to service and repair of the hearing aid would be solved. It would be very easy, without further surgery required. The only 'internal' part would be the piezoelectric ceramic bimorph, its suspension and the wires.

A second possibility is illustrated in figure 2. As mentioned above working on the stapes always includes a risk of inducing a permanent cochlear damage. The risk of adverse reactions of foreign material in the middle ear in patients with chronic ear disease should also be kept in mind. By placing a titanium screw in the solid angle region in the mas-

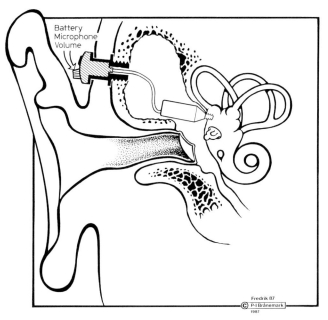

Fig. 2. Schematic drawing of a transducer anchored in or close to the otic capsule. Battery, microphone and volume control are on a percutaneous coupling.

toid cavity a good anchorage for a piezoelectric transducer ought to be able to achieve. This transducer, including a counterweight, would not need any further support but just some leads to an osseo-integrated titanium screw equipped with a percutaneous coupling. However, the optimal mode of vibrations must be studied, which could probably be done using the laser Doppler principle.

Conclusion

The use of mechanical stimuli in order to amplify sound is one way to help patients with impaired hearing. Further knowledge of the properties of vibration in the mastoid and the otic capsule is important and studies regarding these problems with laser Doppler technique are essential. By using the knowledge and experience concerning piezoelectric bimorphs for middle ear implants and percutaneous connectors a new concept in the field of hearing aids could be introduced.

References

1 Brånemark, P.-I.; Hansson, B.-O.; Adell, R.; Reine, U.J.; Hallén, O.; Öhman, A.: Osseointegrated implants in the treatment of edentulous jaw. Scand. J. plast. reconstr. Surg. *11:* suppl. 16 (1977).

2 Adell, R.; Lekholm, U.; Rockler, B.; Brånemark, P.-I.: A fifteen year study of osseointegrated implants in the treatment of the edentulous jaw. Int. J. oral Surg. *10:* 387 (1981).

3 Albrektsson, T.; Brånemark, P.-I.; Hansson, A.-H.; Lindström, J.: Osseointegrated titanium implants. Acta orthop. scand. *52:* 155–170 (1981).

4 Tjellström, A.; Rosenhall, U.; Lindström, J.; Hallén, O.; Albrektsson, I.; Brånemark, P.-I.: Five-years experience with skin-penetrating bone-anchored implants in the temporal bone. Acta oto-lar., Stockh. *95:* 568–575 (1983).

5 Albrektsson, T.; Brånemark, P.-I.; Hansson, A.-H.; Kasemo, B.; Larsson, K.; Lundström, I.; McQueen, D.H.; Skalak, R.: The interface zone of inorganic implants in vivo: titanium implants in bone. Ann. biomed. Eng. *11:* 1–27 (1983).

6 Albrektsson, T.: The response of bone to titanium implants. CRC crit. Rev. Biocompat. *1:* 53–84 (1985).

7 Tjellström, A.: Percutaneous implants in clinical practice. CRC crit. Rev. Biocompat. *1:* 205–228 (1985).

8 Tjellström, A.; Yontchev, E.; Lindström, J.; Brånemark, P.-I.: Five years experience with bone-anchored auricular prostheses. Oto-laryngol. Head Neck Surg. *93:* 366–372 (1985).

9 Kasemo, B.; Lausmaa, J.: Metal selection and surface characteristics; in Brånemark, Tissue-integrated prostheses. Osseointegration in clinical dentistry, pp. 99–116, (Quintessence Press, Chicago 1985).

10 Brånemark, P.-I.: Introduction to osseointegration; in Brånemark, Tissue-integrated prostheses. Osseointegration in clinical dentistry, pp. 11–76 (Quintessence Press, Chicago 1985).

11 Albrektsson, T.; Brånemark, P.-I.; Jacobsson, M.; Tjellström, A.: Present clinical applications of osseointegrated percutaneous implants. Plastic reconstr. Surg., vol. 79, *5:* 721–730 (1987).

12 Holgers, K.M.; Tjellström, A.; Bjursten, L.M.; Erlandsson, B.E.: Soft tissue reactions around percutaneous implants: a clinical study on skin-penetrating titanium implants used for bone-anchored auricular prostheses. Int. J. oral maxillofac. implants, vol. 2, *1:* 35–39 (1987).

13 Suzuki, J.; Kodera, K.; Yanagihara, N.: Evaluation of middle-ear implant: a six month observation in cats. Acta oto-lar. *95:* 646–650 (1983).

14 Yanagihara, N.; Yamanaka, E.; Gyo, K.: Implantable hearing aid using an ossicular vibrator composed of a piezoelectric ceramic bimorph: application to four patients. Am. J. Otol. *8:* 213–219 (1987).

Anders Tjellström, MD, PhD, Department of Otolaryngology,
Sahlgren's Hospital, University of Göteborg, S-413 45 Göteborg (Sweden)

Technical Aspect

Adv. Audiol., vol. 4, pp. 51–72 (Karger, Basel 1988)

Structure and Performance of the Main Components

Tohru Ohno[a], Takeshi Kajiya[a], Hajime Miura[b]

[a] Rion Co., Ltd., Tokyo; [b] Electrotechnical Laboratory, Agency of
Industrial Science and Technology, Tsukuba, Japan

Vibrator

In order to develop a middle ear implant (MEI) with low power consumption and high driving efficiency, it is essential to choose a driving
region which transmits vibration most effectively to the cochlea. Various
locations, such as the head of the stapes, round window, were examined
as to their suitability. The solution chosen as a result of intensive research was to implant the vibrator at the stapes head, as this area has
high vibrational sensitivity and is surgically safe. In the tympanic cavity,
where the head of the stapes is located, space is limited. Therefore, the vibrator should be as small as possible and its construction must permit
easy mounting. As the vibrator will be exposed to high humidity in the
tympanic cavity for several years, outstanding reliability is essential, and
it must be biocompatible to prevent inflammation [Suzuki et al., 1980;
Shono et al., 1983]. Further requirements are low electrical power consumption combined with high output displacement. The power consumption of the vibrator has a direct bearing on the life or the size of the battery for the totally implantable MEI (T-MEI).

The sensitivity of the vibrator defined as the output displacement for
a given input signal is an important consideration which determines the
maximum output level of the MEI and the suitable application range for
patients.

The above is a short outline of the conditions and requirements concerning the vibrator. Several of these requirements stand in inverse relation to each other. To find the optimum solution, various vibrator princi-
ples were considered, such as electromagnetic, moving coil or piezoelec-

tric types. The decision was finally made for a piezoelectric ceramic vibrator, as this type permits easy miniaturization and has low power consumption. The vibrator element is a bimorph design consisting of two narrow hot-pressed ceramic strips (thickness 0.2 mm, width 1.4 mm). Three different types with a length of 5, 7 or 9 mm are provided, to accommodate the individual requirements of patients. The element surface consists of biocompatible materials, and the lead wires are coated with fluoroplastic resin.

When the vibrator is implanted in the tympanic cavity, the distance between the temporal bone and the bone wall of the tympanic cavity, as well as the relative placement of the fulcrum attached to the tympanic cavity wall and the head of the stapes must be critically adjusted by means of a suitable mounting mechanism for the vibrator element. Rion has developed two mounting structures [Shono et al., 1983], as shown in figure 1, which can be selected depending on surgical requirements.

With the double-sliding type shown in figure 1a [Yanagihara et al., 1983], the horizontal distance between the temporal fixing plate and the head of the stapes can be adjusted by moving the sliding plate horizontally in relation to the fixing plate. The sliding cylinder can be moved vertically in relation to the fixing pole, thereby controlling the height from the temporal surface to the fulcrum supported by the wall of the tympanic cavity. The fixed edge of the vibrator element is held by mounting adjustors, and the height from the vibrator tip to the head of the stapes can be adjusted by moving the outer section of the sliding cylinder. The position of the moving parts is fixed by adhesive after the adjustment.

The supporting plate type shown in figure 1b permits adjustment of the horizontal distance between the temporal fixing plate and the stapes by moving the supporting plate horizontally in relation to the fixing plate. The vertical distance between the temporal surface and the head of the stapes and the angle between the bimorph element and the stapes is adjusted by bending the neck of the supporting plate. With both types, a platinum wire or a ceramic cap are attached to the free edge of the vibrator to transmit the vibration to the stapes. These parts are joined to the stapes by the growth of biological tissue.

With a given battery voltage, the sensitivity of the vibrator (output displacement vs. input signal voltage) directly determines the maximum output of the MEI. Therefore, high sensitivity is desirable. In order to yield increased sensitivity, the bimorph element should be as thin and as long as possible. To be implantable in the tympanic cavity, the element

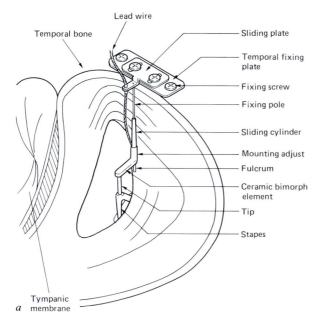

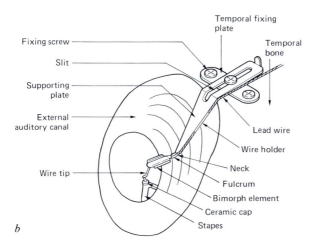

Fig. 1. Vibrator mounting. *a* Double-sliding type. *b* Supporting-plate type.

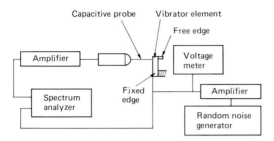

Fig. 2. Displacement measurement set-up.

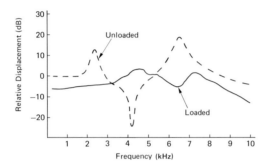

Fig. 3. Simulated frequency response of the vibrator.

length will usually be around 7 mm, and therefore a reduction in thickness is desirable. This parameter, however, is limited by several other factors, such as handling during the operation and resistance to shock. To prolong the life of the vibrator after implanting, electrical insulation should be high, which can be achieved by using a thicker insulation layer.

However, this in turn will reduce sensitivity. The following target parameters were finally selected after intensive discussion of all the aspects mentioned above. Thickness of bimorph element: 0.4 mm or more, insulation after 2 years of implantation: 5 MΩ or more, output level for a 1,000 Hz 1 V_{p-p} input: equivalent to 90 dB SPL or more by tympanic membrane conversion.

The physical amplitude-frequency response was measured using a prototype noncontact measuring system [Shono et al., 1983], as shown in figure 2. For the measurement, a random noise signal was fed to the vibrator and a capacitive probe was placed in close vicinity of the free edge

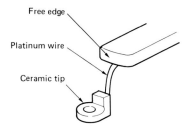

Fig. 4. Platinum and ceramic tip attached to the free edge of the vibrator in animal experiments.

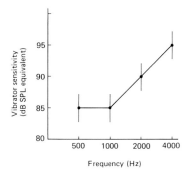

Fig. 5. Tympanic membrane converted sound pressure level (SPL) of ABR test when a 1 Vp-p signal is applied to 5 mm vibrator attached to cat stapes.

of the vibrator element. The ratio between the signal voltage applied to the vibrator and the mechanical displacement amplitude of the free edge, as detected by the capacitive probe, was examined with a spectrum analyzer for each frequency. The results of this test are shown in figure 3. The broken line indicates the unloaded response of the free edge of the vibrator and the solid line shows the response when a simulated load approximately corresponding to the mechanical impedance of the stapes and the inner ear is coupled to the free edge of the vibrator. The response in the loaded condition is approximately flat. The attenuation of about 6 dB in relation to the unloaded curve shows that the mechanical impedance matching is ideal. When the vibrator was loaded to the stapes and inner ear of a live cat, the amplitude-frequency response became even flatter.

The tympanic-membrane-converted sensitivity-frequency response was determined by animal experiments and clinical trials. For this purpose, a platinum wire and ceramic tip were attached to the free edge of the vibrator (figure 4). The animal experiments [Kodera et al., 1981; Kodera and Suzuki, 1981] were conducted with cats. A detailed explanation of the test procedure is contained in part III of this book. The results are shown in figure 5. The tympanic-membrane-converted sound pressure level [Araki et al., 1981] when a signal of 1 V_{p-p} was applied to a 5 mm vibrator was 85 dB at 1,000 Hz, and 95 dB at 4,000 Hz. The results of tests with cats conducted by Guinan and Peake [1967] are shown in figure 6. These curves show the stapedial amplitude characteristics for cats with identical sensation levels. Considering the fact that the physical displacement-frequency response is approximately flat, it may be said that the results gained through our research closely match those of Guinan and Peake.

The clinical tests [Yanagihara et al., 1983] were conducted on volunteer patients who were operated on for chronic tympanitis and facial paralysis. The test procedure is also explained in part III and therefore need not be described here. The vibrator sensitivity, as determined with pure-tone thresholds of hearing tests, is shown in table I and figure 7 [Shaw, 1962]. The signal voltage here is given as an effective (rms) value, in order to permit easy evaluation of the MEI performance. The following relation exists between the peak-to-peak value used in figure 5 and the rms value:

$$V_{rms} = \frac{V_{p-p}}{2\sqrt{2}}$$

The sound quality of the vibrator was also evaluated by means of animal and clinical tests. Figure 8 shows the input-output responses of a vibrator attached to the stapes and an earphone of a behind-the-ear (BTE) type hearing aid attached to the external auditory canal of a cat. Tone pips were used as input signals, and the vibrational waveform was measured with a capacitive probe. The acoustic waveform of the tympanic membrane of the earphone was determined by means of a probe microphone. The output waveform of the earphone shows ringing at decay time. The same effect was observed when measuring the vibration of the long process of the incus with a capacitive probe. The vibrator response, on the other hand, is faithful to the input signal. This suggests that the sound quality, when using a vibrator, will be experienced as natural and clear with words which have a sudden rise and decay, as tone pips.

This expectation was clearly proven by the clinical tests [Yanagihara et al., 1983]. The speech sound list used for speech discrimination tests

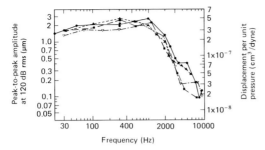

Fig. 6. Stapes amplitude characteristics for cats with identical sensation levels. Middle ear transfer characteristics for the 4 cats on which measurements were made at the largest number of frequencies. It took between 12 and 32 h to take the data for each cat. For cat 30, the decrease in amplitude from the beginning to the end of the experiment is indicated by the two dots at 300 Hz. In this case, the readings were taken 16 h apart. ▽ = cat 19; ■ = cat 20; ▲ = cat 28; ● = cat 30 (from Guinan and Peake, 1967).

Table I. Tympanic membrane conversion sound pressure level with human ear 1 V_{rms} signal is applied at various frequencies

Element length, mm	Capacity, pF	Frequency, Hz						
		250	500	1,000	2,000	3,000	4,000	6,000
5	1,050	89	89	94	103	107	109	110
7	1,550	93	93	98	107	111	113	114
9	1,950	97	97	102	109	113	115	115

Sensitivity deflection: ± 3 dB.

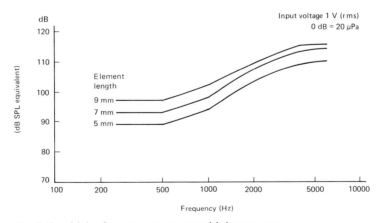

Fig. 7. Sensitivity-frequency response with human ear.

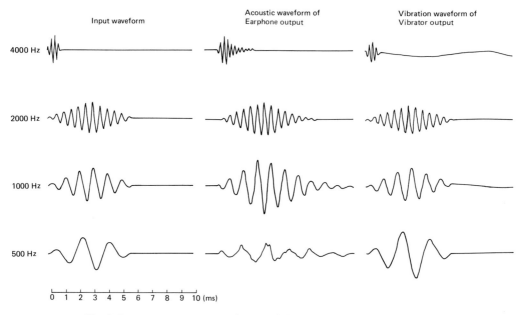

Fig. 8. Input-output response characteristics.

was fed into an audiometer, and the output of the audiometer was connected to a vibrator in contact with the stapes of patients. Approximately the same speech discrimination score was achieved as before the operation [Gyo et al., 1982]. The sound quality as heard through the vibrator was described by patients with remarks such as 'utterly natural', 'sound is clearer than when heard through hearing aid', 'sound does not have a "mechanical" quality', 'I never knew music was so beautiful', etc. [Gyo et al., 1983].

The estimation of how many years an implanted vibrator would remain functional without degradation was very difficult, as no relevant previous data exist. After gathering many data in general reliability tests and considering and thoroughly comparing various methods, the following accelerated life test [Shono et al., 1983] was adopted. The vibrator is placed in a saline solution at 80 °C and a DC voltage of 3 V is applied. The acceleration factor is taken as 40, which corresponds to implanting of the device in a body at a temperature of 40 °C. The electrical insulation of the vibrator after manufacture is in the order of several tens of megohms. As the output impedance of the amplifier used in the totally implantable MEI is comparatively high (about 500 kΩ), the predicted life expectancy point was defined as the point at which the insulation resistance fell below 5 MΩ. This test yielded a life expectancy of over 3 years. With a partially implantable MEI (P-MEI), the vibrator is driven by an inner coil with a much lower impedance (5 kΩ) and is not subject to DC voltage, therefore the vibrator life can be expected to be longer than that of the T-MEI.

External Component of the P-MEI

The external component of the P-MEI supplies the electrical speech signal to the vibrator by means of a link coil. The construction of the external component is shown in figure 9. Basically, it resembles a BTE hearing aid with an integrated outer coil instead of the output earphone. The external component must be adjustable over a wide range to suit the individual bone-conduction hearing acuity of patients with an implanted vibrator and inner coil. Therefore, the external component possesses a tone control, a noise suppressor, a subgain control and an automatic gain control (AGC). Figure 10 shows the block diagram and figure 11 the dimensions and external appearance of the external component. As two frequency response characteristics are provided for the upper frequency range, the tone control circuit is designed for continuously adjustable response in the low range only. The frequency response [Shono et al., 1983] as measured at the output terminal of the inner coil is shown in figure 12.

When the switch of the external component is set to 'S', the noise suppressor is activated, producing the response [Shono et al., 1983] shown in figure 13. This serves to reduce environment noise, whose spectrum is usually concentrated in the frequency range below 500 Hz. The gain control is made up of the subgain control with a 12 dB adjustment range and the main gain control with a 30 dB adjustment range. The subgain control is preadjusted to suit the hearing level of the patient, while the regular gain control can be used by the patient himself to adjust the gain in accordance to the intensity of the external sound picked up by the microphone. Figure 14 [Shono et al., 1983] shows the full-on gain at the inner coil output vs. the input sound pressure level at the microphone when adjusting the subgain control. In order to account for the thickness of the skin between the outer and inner coil, the measurement was performed with a clearance of 5.7 mm between the respective coil housings.

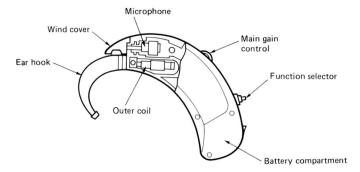

Fig. 9. Construction of external component.

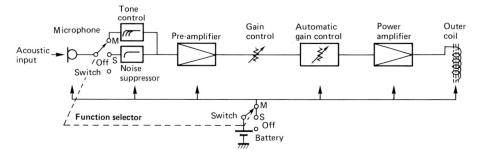

Fig. 10. Block diagram of external component.

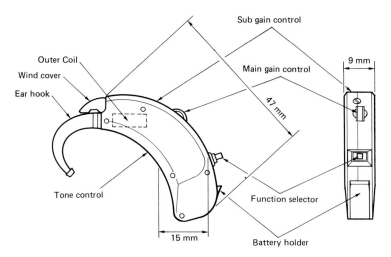

Fig. 11. Outward appearances and dimension of the outside component.

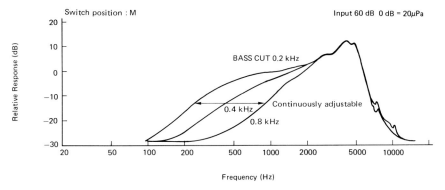

Fig. 12. Tone control characteristics.

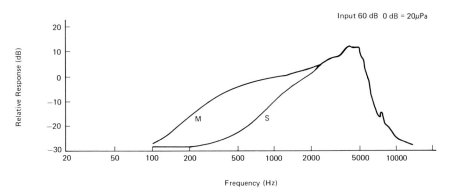

Fig. 13. Noise suppressor characteristics.

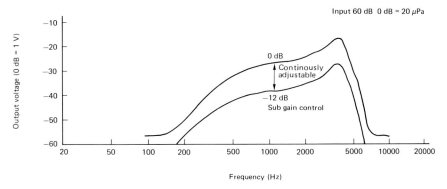

Fig. 14. Full-on gain of external component.

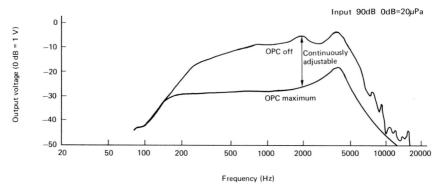

Fig. 15. Output saturation level of external component.

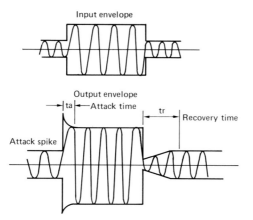

Fig. 16. Transient response of the AGC.

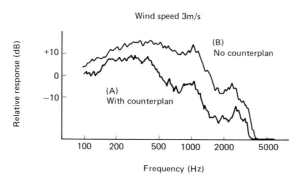

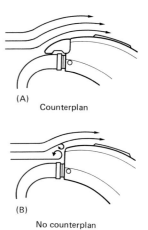

Fig. 17. Efficacy of the wind noise counterplan.

Table II. Specifications of external component

Maximum gain	−28 ±3 dB/V (input 60 dB SPL)
Maximum output level (input 90 dB SPL)	
Peak value	less than −1 dB/V (typ. −4 dB/V)
Average	−9 ±3 dB/V
500 Hz	−11 dB/V
Tone control	Bass-cut continuous
Maximum output noise	less than −51 dB/V (typ. −57 dB/V)
Total harmonic distortion	
500 Hz	less than 2% (typ. 0.8%)
800 Hz	less than 2% (typ. 0.8%)
1,600 Hz	less than 1% (typ. 0.5%)
Output limiting system	AGC limiting 0 to −18 dB continuous attack time less than 10 ms (typ. 3 ms) recovery time less than 150 ms (typ. 100 ms)
Gain control	main control 30 db/subgain control 12 dB continuous
Battery current	less than 2.2 mA (typ. 1.8 mA)
Battery life	142 h (A675), 90 h (675 P)
Dimensions	47×15×9 mm
Weight (without battery)	6.4 g

For the AGC the AGC-limiting principle (OPC) was chosen, as it results in low distortion also when the output is compressed. The compressed output level is continuously variable over a range of 18 dB, as shown in figure 15. The attack time of the output envelope (figure 16) is less than 10 ms, with a typical value of 3 ms, and the recovery time is less than 150 ms, with a typical value of 100 ms. The function of the automatic gain control is to protect the hearing aid from sudden loud noises picked up by the microphone and to prevent amplifying such noises to the uncomfortable loudness level. The circuit also prevents discomfort when the aided patient himself speaks with a loud voice. The external component of the P-MEI is supported by an ear hook on the auricle. The front section of the microphone is protected by a wind cover and wind screen, to minimize wind noise during outdoor use. The effect of the wind noise counterplan is shown in figure 17 [Shono et al., 1983]. The specifications of the external component are shown in table II.

Table III. Specifications of inner coil

Output impedance	5 kΩ (1,000 Hz)
Sensitivity	−78 dB/10 mA/m (1,000 Hz)
Dimensions	37.5×25×7.2 mm
Volume	6.3 cm³
Weight	9.3 g

was performed with a clearance of 5.7 mm between the housings of the inner coil and the external coil.

The canceling effect produced by the canceling coil was 55 dB in a uniform magnetic field. At a distance of about 1 m from the source of the field, the effect was 20 to 30 dB, which should pose no problem when the unit is used under ordinary conditions.

An accelerated life prediction test [Shono et al., 1983] was carried out by placing the inner coil in a normal saline solution of 80 °C and applying a DC voltage of 3 V. The acceleration factor was taken as 40, and the predicted life expectancy point was defined as the point at which the insulation between the normal saline solution and the inner coil terminals fell below 5 MΩ. This test, which may be considered more demanding than conditions of actual use, yielded a life expectancy of over 3 years. The specifications of the inner coil are shown in table III.

Implantable Connector

This connector was developed to connect the lead wires of implanted components, and to serve as a terminal board from which the lead wires are disconnected when components are replaced. The connector is useful also for checking purposes if a component should break down, and for the transition from the P-MEI to the T-MEI.

The connector construction (figure 21) [Shono et al., 1983] ensures that the connection and removal of wires, as well as filling and tear-out of insulation material can be carried out easily during the operation. The connector case is made of polypropylene resin and consists of the lid and an integrated hinge. The terminal screws are fixed to a base plate of methaacrylic resin which is fitted in the bottom of the connector. The lead wires are inserted in the fixing slits and fastened to the terminals by means

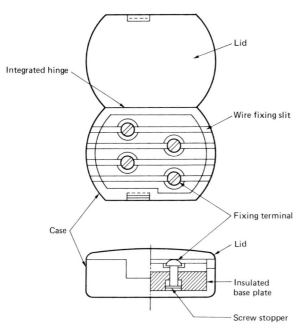

Fig. 21. Implantable connector.

of the screws. Then the connector is filled with silicone resin and the lid, which possesses an under-cut claw, is closed. This process can be carried out in approximately 10 min. The life expectancy of the connector, as determined with an accelerated life prediction test in the same way as described above, was established to be more than 3 years. The connector dimensions are $18 \times 12 \times 6$ mm, the volume is 1 cm^3, and the weight 1.6 g.

Implantable Microphone

The microphone for the T-MEI is designed to be implanted below the skin of the external auditory canal. Small dimensions and high sensitivity are important prerequisites for such a microphone, and high reliability is also essential to ensure steady long-term operation in vivo. Therefore, an electret condenser microphone was chosen as a transducer, as the sensitivity of this type of microphone does not decrease with size. The microphone is hermetically enclosed in a metal capsule together with the FET used to convert the output impedance to a lower value.

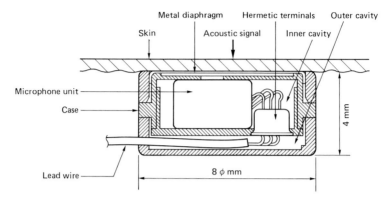

Fig. 22. Structure of the implantable microphone.

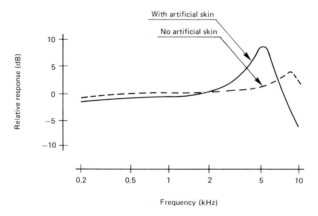

Fig. 23. Frequency response of the implantable microphone.

The structure of the implantable microphone is shown in figure 22 [Araki et al., 1983]. The microphone unit contains the microphone and FET and measures 3.5×3.5×2.3 mm. The capsule is made of stainless steel (SUS 316L) and divided into an inner and an outer cavity. Sound vibrations are transmitted to the wall of the inner cavity through the skin. To prevent biological fluid from entering the cavity, the 9 μm vibrating membrane made of stainless steel (SUS 316L) is laser-welded [Kodera and Suzuki, 1981]. The electrical output signal of the FET is supplied to the lead wires in the outer cavity via the hermetic terminals. The inner

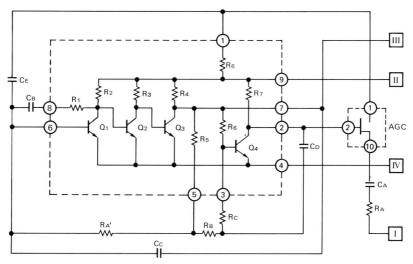

Fig. 24. Circuit of the implantable amplifier.

Table IV. Final specifications of the implantable amplifier

Working voltage	1.2 to 1.5 V
Current consumption	20 to 25 μA
Input impedance	1.8 kΩ (at maximum gain)
Voltage gain	48 dB (1,000 Hz N characteristic at max. gain)
Output impedance	15 kΩ
No distortion maximum output	
voltage	0.27 to 0.28 V
Inner noise level	less than 3 μV (input converted)
Automatic gain controler	working input Level 90 dB SPL
Frequency response	100 to 5,000 Hz – 4 dB (N-characteristic)
	6 dB/octave adjustable (L-characteristic)

cavity is filled with argon gas to prevent oxidation, and the outer cavity is filled with epoxy resin to protect the electrical insulation of the lead wires connected to the hermetic terminals. The outside of the microphone is coated with a 5-μm layer of polyxylylene resin to improve encapsulation by the biological tissue. The outer diameter of the entire unit is 8 mm, and its thickness is 4 mm.

When operated with a battery voltage of 0.7–1.1 V, the electrical current consumption of the implantable microphone is 20–30 μA. The output impedance is 2.4–2.8 kΩ, and the sensitivity at 1,000 Hz when con-

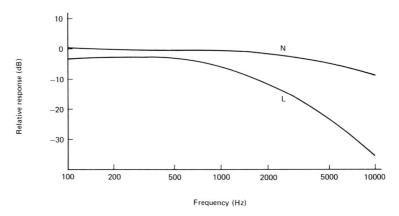

Fig. 25. Frequency response of the implantable amplifier.

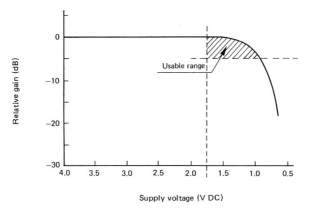

Fig. 26. Effect of supply voltage variation on gain of the implantable amplifier.

nected to a 5 kΩ load is –54 dB (0 dB relative 1 V/Pa). The noise level is 1.5 to 3 μV (input converted), corresponding to 33 dB(A). The frequency response, as shown by the broken line in figure 23 [Araki et al., 1983], is almost flat from 200 to 5,000 Hz. When artificial skin (made from natural gum and silicon grease) with a thickness of 1 mm is placed on the vibrating membrane, the sensitivity at 1,000 Hz decreases by 1 dB, and the frequency response becomes as shown by the solid line in figure 23. The accelerated life prediction test carried out under the same conditions as for the vibrator and inner coil yielded a life expectancy of more than 3 years.

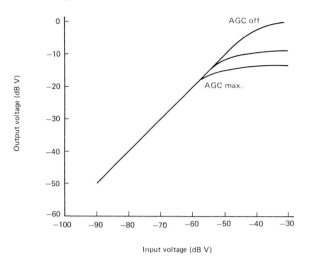

Fig. 27. Input-output response of the implantable amplifier.

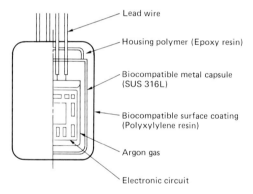

Fig. 28. Structure of the implantable amplifier.

Implantable Amplifier

The amplifier for the T-MEI must have a low electric current consumption and a high reliability. The operating voltage and current consumption must be on the same order as for the microphone to permit parallel as well as in-series connection, and the inherent noise level should be low. The design target values were voltage gain 50 dB, frequency range 200 to 5,000 Hz, input-converted inherent noise level below 3 μV, and automatic gain control (AGC) as sound-processing circuit.

After repeated tests and experiments, the hybrid integrated circuit shown in figure 24 was chosen; it consists of a discrete amplifier and an AGC circuit [Shono et al., 1983]. Table IV shows the final specifications of the amplifier. The frequency response is shown in figure 25, and the effect of supply voltage variations on the gain of the amplifier are seen in figure 26. The input–output response of the AGC circuit is plotted in figure 27. As can be seen from figure 28, the construction of the implantable amplifier [Shono et al., 1983] resembles that of the inner coil. The housing dimensions are $6.5 \times 13.5 \times 23.5$ mm. The accelerated life prediction test carried out under the same conditions as for the other implantable components yielded a life expectancy of more than 3 years.

Tohru Ohno, Rion Co., Ltd., Kokubunji Tokyo 185 (Japan)

Adv. Audiol., vol. 4, pp. 73–84 (Karger, Basel 1988)

Energy Source for the Middle Ear Implant

Hironosuke Ikeda[a], *Nobuhiro Furukawa*[a], *Satoru Narukawa*[a], *Shiro Yoshizawa*[b]

[a] Sanyo Electric Co., Ltd., Osaka; [b] Faculty of Engineering, Kyoto University, Kyoto, Japan

Introduction

Several hundred thousands persons are using pacemakers in the world. The typical implantable power sources for cardiac pacemakers are iodine lithium cells and silver chromate lithium cells. As biotechnology has progressed rapidly and as the proportion of elderly people is increasing, the demand for implantable equipment and power sources for this equipment should increase more and more.

In this chapter we describe the results achieved from 1978 to 1983 with the support of the Ministry of International Trade and Industry in the development of power sources for middle ear implants (MEI).

Two types of cell for MEI have been developed. One is the nonrechargeable primary battery and the other is the rechargeable secondary battery. The tested results of the small size batteries are shown in table I.

From those results, zinc-air cells have the high energy density of 860 Wh/l. This cell reaction, which requires oxygen in air, is represented by the following equation:

$$\tfrac{1}{2} O_2 + Zn \rightarrow ZnO$$

then this zinc-air cell is not suitable as a power source for the MEI.

$I_2(PVP)/Li$ cells are now used as a power source for cardiac pacemakers. But $I_2(PVP)/LI$ cells use a solid electrolyte which cannot give sufficient current as a power source for an MEI, because of the high resistance of the cell. The driving current of the MEI is higher than that of a cardiac pacemaker. Ag_2CrO_4/Li cells have the high energy density of 570 Wh/l. This cell reaction is represented by the following equation:

$$2Li + Ag_2CrO_4 \rightarrow Li_2CrO_4 + 2Ag.$$

Table I. Specifications of small size batteries

Cell	System	Voltage V	Energy density	
			WH/l	WH/kg
Mercury cell	HgO/Zn	1.35	450	100
Nickel-zinc cell	NiOOH/Zn	1.6	225	70
Alkaline manganese cell	Alk, MnO_2/Zn	1.5	160	50
Zinc-air cell	Air/Zn	1.3	860	250
Silver oxide cell	Ag_2O/Zn	1.55	390	120
Manganese dioxide lithium cell	MnO_2/Li	3.0	510	170
Silver chromate lithium cell	Ag_2CrO_4/Li	3.1	570	190
Graphite-fluoride lithium cell	(CF)n/Li	3.0	375	120
Iodine-lithium solid cell	I_2(PVP)/Li	2.8	710	230

In this cell reaction, the products are generated in two phases, i.e. silver metal and lithium chromate. This means that the reaction products grow and the cell expands. Therefore, this cell is also unsuitable as a power source for the MEI. MnO_2/Li have the high energy density of 510 Wh/l and the high voltage of 3.0 V. The mechanism of the electrode reaction is the diffusion in solid phase represented by the following equation:

$$Li + Mn^{4+}O_2 \rightarrow Mn^{3+} (Li).$$

The product of this reaction is monophase and the expansion of the positive electrode is small. The operating voltage is 3.0 V instead of 1.5 V. Considering this point, MnO_2/Li cell was selected for MEI.

We investigated some systems of small secondary batteries as well. The small secondary batteries are usually nickel-cadmium, nickel-zinc or secondary silver batteries. Nickel-zinc and silver batteries have a high energy density, but do not have a long cycle life. The performances of these batteries on overcharge and overdischarge are not as good as those of the nickel-cadmium cell. We selected the nickel-cadmium cell as the secondary power source of MEI in view of its good cycle performance and stability for overcharge and overdischarge. The secondary battery is implanted in the body and recharged by means of an electromagnetic induction method for safety and certainty. The equipment for the electromagnetic induction method basically consists of two iron cores and coils. The primary coil is placed in the charger and the secondary coil is placed in the battery.

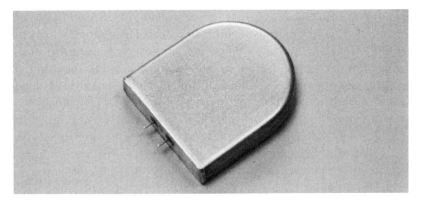

Fig. 1. External appearance of secondary power source.

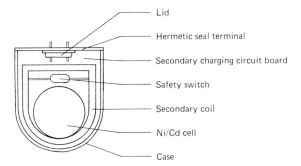

Fig. 2. Internal construction of secondary power source.

Secondary Battery

Construction

The external appearance of the secondary power source is shown in figure 1, its internal appearance in figure 2. The secondary power source is composed of a nickel-cadmium cell, a secondary charging circuit and a safety apparatus. The specification of the secondary power source is shown in table II.

Nickel-Cadmium Cell

As this nickel-cadmium cell is going to be implanted in the living body, it must have high reliability and good performance under the conditions of the body temperature and high humidity. Therefore, highly re-

Table II. Specifications of secondary power source

Model	J-KB-03
Cell system	sealed Ni/Cd secondary cell
Dimensions	21(W) × 23.5(L) × 5.3(T) mm
Case material	stainless steel
Sealing method	hermetic seal by laser-welding
Helium leak rate	less than 9×10^{-9} atm · cm^3/s
Weight	about 5.5 g
Voltage	1.2 V
Capacity	more than 20 mAh
Cycle life	over 2 years
Internal impedance	less than 500 Ω (1.2 V 50 μA)
Safety mechanism	emergency cut-off circuit (cut-off by magnet)
Operating temperature	body temperature

liable electrode constitutions and cell constructions were investigated. Considering implantable battery space and operation time for one charge, a button cell of 12.5 mm in diameter and 3.5 mm in height was adopted. This battery can drive on MEI for 2 weeks with one charge.

Battery Seal Construction. A ceramic seal was selected for the hermetic sealing of the cell. The internal construction of the hermetically sealed nickel-cadmium button cell is shown in figure 3.

Positive Electrode. A sintered nickel electrode is adopted in view of reliability.

Negative Electrode. A pressed cadmium electrode is adopted because of its larger capacity and better charge-discharge characteristics at high temperature than those of the sintered cadmium electrode. The pressed cadmium electrode is mainly composed of the mixture of CdO, Cd powder and other compounds.

Acceleration cycle performance is over 300 cycles at body temperature. This number of cycles corresponds to about 10 years of operation of an MEI.

Electrolyte. Generally, when a potassium hydroxide solution is used as the electrolyte, the charge-discharge characteristics are good at room temperature, but not so at high temperatures. In order to find an electrolyte with superior characteristics at body temperature, the kind and com-

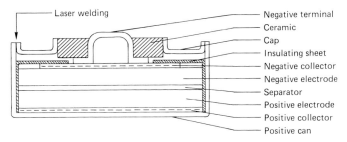

Fig. 3. Internal construction of hermetically sealed Ni/Cd button cell.

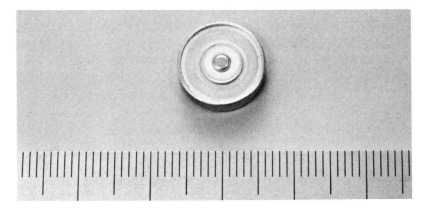

Fig. 4. External appearance of complete battery.

position of electrolytes were examined. A potassium hydroxide solution added with sodium hydroxide and lithium hydroxide was found to be suitable.

The Complete Battery. The external appearance of the complete battery is shown in figure 4. Finally, the sintered nickel electrode is used as the positive electrode, the pressed cadmium electrode is used as the negative electrode, the potassium hydroxide solution added with sodium hydroxide and lithium hydroxide is used as the electrolyte and heat-resisting nonwoven fabric is used as the separator. The cell is hermetically sealed and measures 12.5 mm in diameter and 3.5 mm in height. The charge-discharge characteristics of the secondary power source are shown in figure 5.

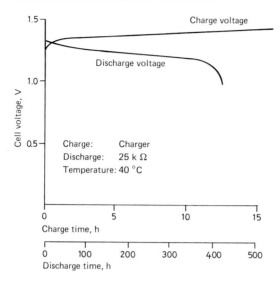

Fig. 5. Charge-discharge characteristics of secondary power source.

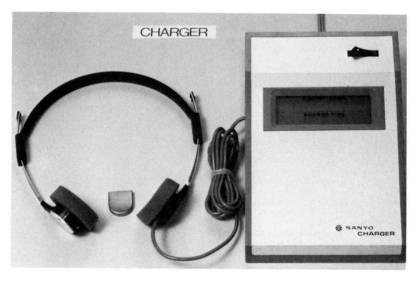

Fig. 6. External appearance of charger.

Table III. Specifications of charger

Style	J-KC-03
Form	charger in electromagnetic induction
Power source	AC 50–60 Hz, 100 V
Power consumption	2 W
Size	$130(W) \times 190(L) \times 65(H)$ mm
Weight	about 1 kg
Operating temperature	0–40 °C
Coil cap	6 mm
Charging current	2.5 mA
Charging time	16 h
Frequency	40–50 kHz
Size of charging coil case	$28.5\emptyset \times 13.5(H)$ mm
Control function	
Charge time	level display
Charging cycle	accumulated charging time by electromagnetic counter
Charging end	warning buzzer
Prevention of overcharge	breaking transmission circuit
Detection of proper position	LCD level

Charger

The external appearance of the charger is shown in figure 6. The charger is composed of electromagnetic induction, position controller and detector, overcharge protector and display of charging state. The head band has a small, light high-frequency transformer. The charging state and time are displayed on the front panel of the charger. The warning buzzer sounds at the end of the charge. The specification of the charger is shown in table III.

Primary Cell

A manganese dioxide lithium cell was selected for the MEI on account of its high energy density and long shelf life. The following items are required for the MEI: (1) long life for continuous operation over 2 years; (2) good cell performance at the living body temperature; (3) high resistance to leakage, and (4) low self-discharge. Various cell components and constructions were examined to see whether they satisfied the above requirements.

Cell Shape

The cell sizes are designed considering that the cell capacity should be sufficient for 2 years' continuous operation, which is the target of the power source for the MEI. A thin type cell is required at the initial stage because of its implantable configuration along head skin. Accordingly, the flexible primary sheet cells whose outer case is composed of a laminated metal sheet were designed and examined from the view point of electrode construction and sealing process. Consequently, a laser-welded flexible cell measuring $45 \times 60 \times 1.1$ mm with a hermetic seal terminal was developed. As a result, higher reliability and higher energy density due to an increase in the available capacity paralleled by a decrease in the sealing part were obtained than with the laminated-sheet-type cells. As it was proposed in 1981 that the cell should be packed in the power source capsule with the safety equipment, the advanced rectangular cell with a laser-welded hermetic-seal terminal was designed and constructed.

Cell Components

A pressed manganese dioxide electrode is used as the cathode electrode. Lithium metal is pressed on the collector and connected to the terminal for the anode. Nonwoven polypropylene fabric and a microporous polypropylene film are piled up for the separator. The electrolyte is prepared by dissolving lithium perchlorate into propylenecarbonate.

The Final Constructed Cell

The cell is 23.5 mm in width, 27 mm in height and 5.5 mm in thickness. The terminal cap and the case are hermetically sealed by glass-to-metal laser-welding. The designed cell capacity is over 500 mAh which is

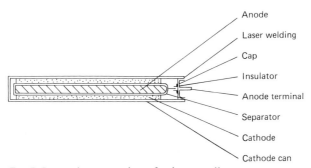

Fig. 7. Internal construction of primary cell.

sufficient to drive the MEI at 25 µA for over 2 years. Cell structure and appearance are shown in figures 7 and 8.

Primary Cell Power Source

The power source is composed of the primary cell and the safety equipment as well as the power source using the secondary cell.

Figure 9 shows the structure of the power source.

Accelerated Test. As it takes very long to measure the cell capacity at usual current of 25 µA (load: 120 kΩ), the accelerated discharge test at 250 µA (load: 12 kΩ) was performed. The result is shown in figure 10. A discharge capacity of over 450 mAh was obtained in 80 days. It was demonstrated that this power source could operate continuously for 2 years, because the capacity of 438 mAh is equal to the discharge capacity at 25 µA for 2 years.

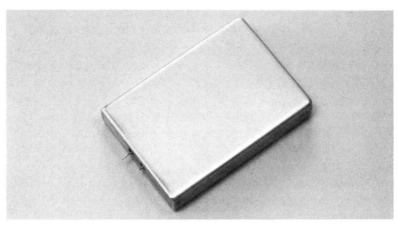

8

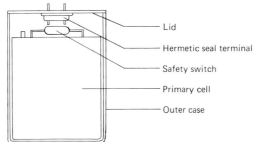

9

Fig. 8. Appearance of primary cell.
Fig. 9. Internal construction of primary power source.

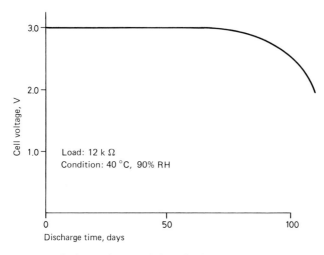

Fig. 10. Discharge characteristics of primary power source.

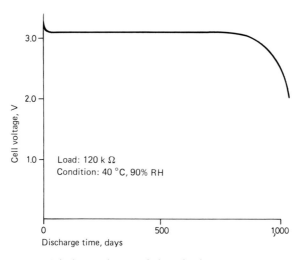

Fig. 11. Discharge characteristics of primary power source.

Discharge Test for Practical Use. The discharge test which was similar to the practical use was examined at a 120-kΩ load (25 µA) at 40 °C, 90% relative humidity (RH), as shown in figure 11.

It was clarified that this power source was suitable as the power source of the MEI, because of its stable discharge voltage of over 3 V.

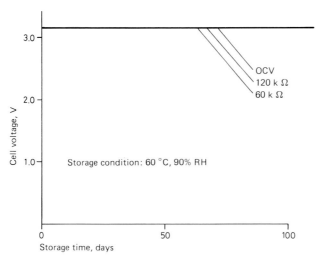

Fig. 12. Storage characteristics of primary power source.

Table IV. Specification of primary power source

Type	J-CB-03
Cell system	manganese dioxide lithium primary cell
Power source size	25.5(W) × 35(H) × 6.2(T) mm
Case material	stainless steel
Sealing	hermetic seal by laser-welding
Helium leak rate	less than 9×10^{-9} atm · cm^3/s (by helium leak detector)
Weight	about 15 g
Voltage	3 V
Capacity	more than 500 mAh
Life	over 2 years
Internal impedance	less than 1000 Ω (3 V, 25 μA)
Safety system	emergency cut circuit by magnet
Operating temperature	body temperature

Storage Test. The changes of the open-circuit voltage and closed-circuit voltage on storage at 60 °C, 90% RH are shown in figure 12. These voltages show no changes. No problem was observed on vibration test and on emergency stop test by the magnet. It was concluded that this power source was suitable for the MEI.

The specification of the developed power source for the MEI is shown in table IV and the appearance in figure 13.

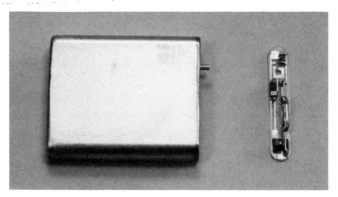

Fig. 13. Appearance of primary power source.

Table V. Achieved performance of power sources

	Target	Achieved
Primary cell (MnO$_2$/Li)		
Energy density	350 mWH/ml	about 400 mWH/ml
Cell life	over 2 years	over 2 years
Cell volume	5 ml (implanted in head)	3.5 ml (capsule only)
	10 ml (implanted in breast)	9.8 ml (including housing)
Secondary cell (Ni/Cd)		
Energy density		about 55 mWH/ml
Cell life	over 2 years	over 2 years
Cell volume	1 ml	0.43 ml (capsule only)
		4.8 ml (including housing)
Charging method	(implanted in the skin of upper part of external auditory meatus or in mastoid process) electromagnetic induction charging or electric wave charging	high frequency electromagnetic induction charging
Charging interval	once a week	once a week

Conclusion

The result is shown in table V. The results demonstrate that the targets for the primary and secondary sources are achieved and that the selected button-type nickel-cadmium cell and manganese-dioxidelithium cell are excellent power sources for the MEI.

H. Ikeda, PhD, Sanyo Electric Co., Moriguchi, Ltd., Osaka 570 (Japan)

Adv. Audiol., vol. 4, pp. 85–96 (Karger, Basel 1988)

Performance of the Middle Ear Implants

Tohru Ohno, Takeshi Kajiya

Rion Co., Ltd., Tokyo, Japan

Performance of the Partially Implantable Middle Ear Implant

The partially implantable MEI (P-MEI) consists of the external component, the inner coil, the implantable connector and the vibrator. It is also possible to directly connect the inner coil and vibrator with lead wires, without using the connector. The block diagram of the P-MEI is shown in figure 1. The outside sounds are picked up by the microphone of the external component and converted into electrical signals. These signals are amplified and processed by the electronic circuits in the external component, and then supplied to the external coil, which generates an electromagnetic field. The electromagnetic flux permeates the skin and induces a signal voltage in the inner coil, which is used to drive the vibrator. The mechanical vibrations are then transmitted as acoustic vibrations to the cochlea.

The clinical experiments in the course of the development program for the MEI and the audiometric measurements on volunteer patients were conducted using an audiometer, and therefore the main measurements were also carried out with pure-tone audiometer test frequencies. However, when evaluating important performance parameters of hearing aids, such as the maximum acoustic gain and the output sound pressure level (SPL) for an input SPL of 90 dB ($OSPL_{90}$), the IEC standard and other regulations prescribe 1,600 Hz or 2,500 Hz. In the following explanation of the level diagrams for each part, 2,000 Hz is used as reference test frequency, and data for other frequencies are shown in the tables or figures.

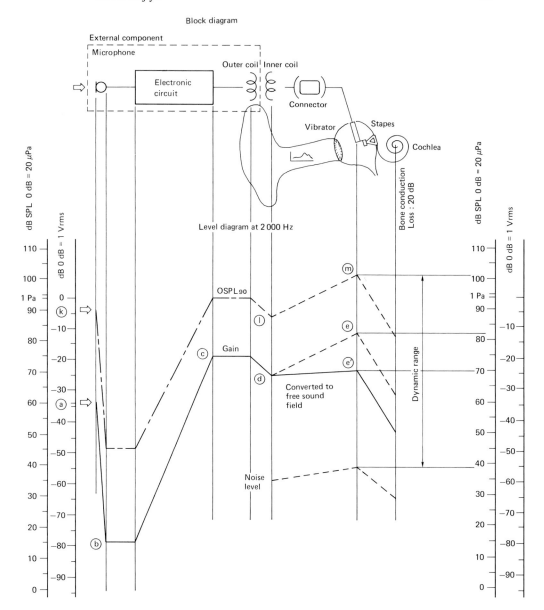

Fig. 1. Block diagram and level diagram of the P-MEI.

Figure 1 also depicts the level diagram [Fukuyama et al., 1983] for the P-MEI when an inner coil with N-characteristics is used. In this example, a sound of 60 dB (fig. 1, a), corresponding to the loudness of a regular speech sound at a distance of 1 m, enters the microphone. The sensitivity of the microphone is −45 dB, with 0 dB defined as the condition when a sound corresponding to 94 dB SPL (0 dB = 20 μPa) produces a 1 volt signal voltage. As the sensitivity of the microphone is −45 dB, a 60 dB input produces the output voltage −45 dB − (94 dB − 60 dB) = −79 dB/V (fig. 1,b). With the gain controls of the amplifier circuits all set to full gain, the voltage gain is 60 dB. The output voltage of the microphone, therefore, is amplified by 60 dB and becomes −79 dB +60 dB = −19 dB/V (fig. 1,c), which is supplied to the outer coil.

When the clearance between the external component and the inner coil housing is 5.7 mm, the transmission loss between the outer and inner coils is 6 dB. Therefore, the voltage −19 db − 6 dB = −25 dB/V (fig, 1,d) is induced in the inner coil. The sensitivity of a vibrator with a 7-mm element is 107 dB. A vibration corresponding to 107 dB −25 dB = 82 dB SPL (fig. 1,e) (tympanic membrane converted) is therefore transmitted by the vibrator to the inner ear. However, as the sound reaching the microphone does not pass through the external auditory canal, the acoustic gain caused by the resonance of this canal is not used, and the sound pressure level difference between the entrance of the external auditory canal in a free sound field and the sound entrance of the microphone must be compensated for. At 2,000 Hz, compensation for the position of the microphone sound entrance is 0 dB, but to compensate for the resonance gain, 12 dB must be subtracted. Therefore the vibration level of the vibrator in the diagram (free field SPL converted) is equivalent to 82 dB −12 dB = 70 dB SPL [Shono et al., 1983] (fig. 1,e).

As outlined above, the input-output gain of the P-MEI at 2,000 Hz is 70 dB −60 dB = 10 dB (free field SPL converted). This amounts to a 10-dB improvement in bone-conduction hearing acuity when such a device is implanted.

Many investigations into the actual gain settings used by hearing aid wearers have revealed that settings at about half the hearing threshold level [Fukuyama et al., 1983], i.e. 30 dB for a patient with a hearing level of 60 dB, are most commonly used. This so-called half-gain rule is presently widely applied in the fitting of hearing aids. It is also said that patients with a mild to moderate hearing impairment tend to use gain set-

Table I. Gain calculation of P-MEI

	Frequencies, Hz						
	250	500	1,000	2,000	3,000	4,000	6,000
Input, SPL (a)				60 dB			
Microphone sensitivity	−45 dB 0 dB = 1 V re 1 Pa (94 dB SPL)						
Microphone output (b) dB re V				−79 dB			
Amplifier plus link coil gain, dB	37	47	51	54	58	61	37
Inner coil output (d) V	−42	−32	−28	−25	−21	−18	−42
Vibrator sensitivity dB SPL re V	93	93	98	107	111	113	114
Tympanic membrane conversion SPL (e), dB	51	61	70	82	90	95	72
Ear canal resonance compensate, dB	− 1	− 2	− 2	−12	−16	−14	−7
Microphone position compensate, dB	− 1	− 1	− 4	0	0	0	0
Substantial output Level-converted sound field (e') dB SPL	49	58	64	70	74	81	65
Gain, dB	−11	− 2	4	10	14	21	5
L-characteristics (relative response to the N-characteristics), dB	0	0	− 2	− 5	− 9	−12	−16
Gain, dB	−11	− 2	2	5	5	9	−11

The letters in parentheses correspond to the same letters in figure 1.

tings which correspond to one third of their hearing level. By applying these empirical results to the fitting of the P-MEI, it can be deducted that this technique is suitable for patients with a bone-conduction hearing level of 20 to 30 dB.

Table I shows the gain calculation process for a P-MEI with N-characteristics and a vibrator of 7 mm length at various frequencies and for each component separately. Data showing the response difference for the L-characteristics are also shown. The gain frequency response curve is shown in figure 2.

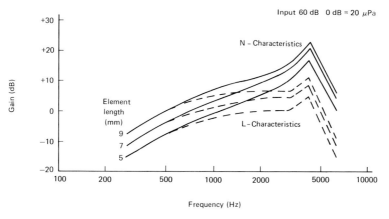

Fig. 2. Gain-frequency response converted to free sound field.

Table II. OSPL$_{90}$ calculation of the P-MEI

	Frequencies, Hz						
	250	500	1,000	2,000	3,000	4,000	6,000
Input SPL (k)				90 dB			
Output level of the inner coil, V	−17	−12	− 9	− 6	− 8	− 4	−19
Vibrator sensitivity dB SPL re V	93	93	98	107	111	113	114
Equivalent OSPL$_{90}$ (m)	76	81	89	101	103	109	95
L-characteristics (relative response to the N-characteristics, dB	0	0	− 2	− 5	− 9	−12	−16
Equivalent OSPL$_{90}$	76	81	87	96	94	97	79

The letters in parentheses correspond to the same letters in figure 1.

Several methods exist to evaluate the maximum output SPL. In this research, tympanic membrane conversion was used, as it permits easy comparison of the OSPL$_{90}$.

When a pure tone with an SPL of 90 dB (fig. 1,k) enters the microphone of the external component, the maximum output voltage of the inner coil at 2,000 Hz is −6 dB re 1 V (fig. 1,l). The vibrator sensitivity at 2,000 Hz is 107 dB. Tympanic membrane conversion results in an OSPL$_{90}$

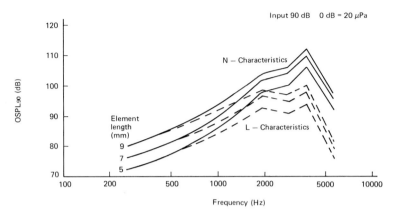

Fig. 3. OSPL$_{90}$ curve.

of 107 dB −6 dB = 101 dB (fig. 1, m) being transmitted to the inner ear. The calculation method for all frequencies is shown in table II and the OSPL$_{90}$ curve in figure 3.

The residual noise level of the P-MEI is determined by the noise level of the microphone, i.e. about −110 dB in terms of output voltage and about 30 dB converted into input SPL. Usually, noise is evaluated at 1,000 Hz. In this case, the noise voltage at the microphone output is amplified by 51 dB in the subsequent stages including the amplifier circuits and the link coil, resulting in −59 dB, which are fed to the vibrator. This noise signal produces a noise vibration which is equivalent to −59 dB +98 dB = 39 dB SPL by tympanic membrane conversion. The dynamic range is defined as the ratio between the maximum output SPL and the noise SPL. A comparison to the equivalent OSPL$_{90}$ data in table II shows that the dynamic range at 1,000 Hz is 50 dB; at 2,000 Hz it is 62 dB, and at 3,000 Hz 64 dB.

When the P-MEI is used by a patient with a bone-conduction hearing loss of 20 dB, as shown in figure 1, the hearing level is improved by about 10 dB, regardless of the air-conduction hearing acuity. In comparison to conventional hearing aids, the P-MEI has several advantages. The air-bone gap is of no consequence, there is no feeling of occlusion as the external auditory canal is not blocked, there is no acoustic feedback, and the tone quality is remarkably good, leading to a high word intelligibility score. In comparison to the totally implantable MEI (T-MEI), there is a cosmetic disadvantage, as the external component can be seen from the outside, but the advantages are that gain and tone quality can be adjusted, a noise suppressor can be used, a higher degree of safety is achieved as the battery is not implanted, and battery replacement is easier to accomplish. As progress in the field of electronics advances, performance improvements will be possible even without changing already implanted components. Therefore, this type of hearing aid promises to become commercially viable.

At the Kitasato Institute, chemical solubility tests were carried out, and the results of injuriousness tests and hemolytic tests were all negative.

Performance of the Totally Implantable Middle Ear Implant

The T-MEI consists of an implantable microphone, an implantable amplifier, a vibrator, an in-the-body-type battery, and an implantable connector. For the battery, the primary type was a lithium-manganese oxide battery; a rechargeable nickel-cadmium battery was also used. As the voltage ratio of these battery types is about 2:1, the implantable microphone and the implantable amplifier were either connected in series or parallel, depending on which battery was used. The performance of the T-MEI was about the same with both batteries, and the following explanation therefore applies to both cases.

The system configuration and the level diagram are shown in figure 4 [Fukuyama et al., 1983]. The difference to the P-MEI is a skin-passing loss of 3 dB, lower microphone sensitivity, an influence of the skin on frequency response, and the fact that the $OSPL_{90}$ is determined by the saturation level of the amplifier. The gain and $OSPL_{90}$ calculation and results are shown in table III, figure 5 and table IV, figure 6.

As with the P-MEI, the residual noise level is -110 dB at the microphone output, -62 dB at the amplifier output, and 36 dB SPL at the vibrator output. Therefore, the dynamic range is 46 dB at 1,000 Hz, 50 dB at 2,000 Hz, and 51 dB at 3,000 Hz.

When compared to conventional hearing aids, the T-MEI has – in addition to the features of the partially implantable MEI – the following qualities. If the emergency switch is not used, it operates also at night, it is invisible from the outside, handling is extremely simple as no gain adjustment or battery replacement by the patient is required, and the patient can use it even for example while diving or at high altitudes (from

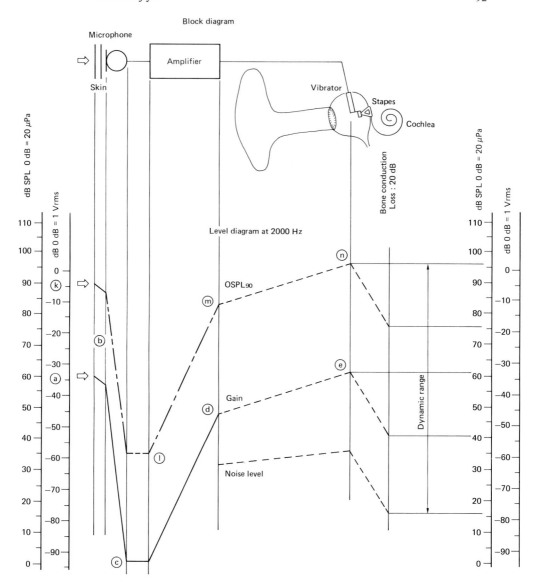

Fig. 4. Block diagram and level diagram of the T-MEI.

Table III. Gain calculation of the T-MEI

	Frequencies, Hz						
	250	500	1,000	2,000	3,000	4,000	6,000
Input SPL (a)				60 dB			
Passing loss of the skin (b)				−3 dB			
Microphone sensitivity (0 dB = 1 V re 1 Pa)	−57	−57	−57	−56	−53	−47	−67
Microphone output (c) dB re V	−94	−94	−94	−93	−90	−84	−104
Amplifier gain, dB	48	48	48	47	46	45	44
Amplifier output (d), dB	−46	−46	−46	46	−44	−39	−60
Vibrator sensitivity dB SPL re V	93	93	98	107	111	113	114
Tympanic membrane conversion SPL (e), dB	47	47	52	61	67	74	54
Gain, dB	−13	−13	− 8	1	7	14	− 6
L-characteristics (relative response to the N-characteristics, dB)	− 2	− 3	− 5	−10	−13	−16	−20
Gain, dB	−15	−16	−13	− 9	− 6	− 2	−26

The letters in parentheses correspond to the same letters in figure 5.

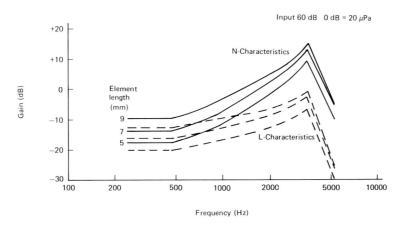

Fig. 5. Gain-frequency response.

Table IV. OSPL$_{90}$ calculation of the T-MEI

	Frequencies, Hz						
	250	500	1,000	2,000	3,000	4,000	6,000
Input level, db SPL				90 dB			
Saturated level of the amplifier output, dB re V				−11 dB			
Vibrator sensitivity dB SPL re V	93	93	98	107	111	113	114
Equivalent OSPL$_{90}$	82	82	87	96	100	102	103
L characteristics (Relative response to the N characteristics) dB	−2	−3	−5	−10	−13	−16	−20
Equivalent OSPL$_{90}$	80	79	82	86	87	86	83

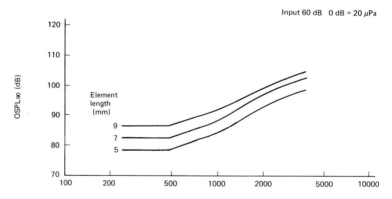

Fig. 6. OSPL$_{90}$ curve.

0.5 to 3 atm). This permits him to lead a completely normal life. The sound-gathering effect of the auricle as well as the resonance effect of the external auditory canal can also be utilized in the same way as for non-aided persons. However, as opposed to the P-MEI, once the T-MEI is implanted, gain or frequency response adjustments are not possible. Other disadvantages are the fact that the life of the vibrator is comparatively short, and the dynamic range is limited. If the primary battery is used, the battery must be exchanged in an operation every 27 months. In case of the rechargeable battery, charging is necessary for an average of about 70 min a day. Due to these difficulties, a commercial realization of the T-MEI is not planned at present.

Efficiency and Future Prospects of the MEI

The gain and maximum output level of MEI at the present stage of development are about equal to bone-conduction hearing aids. The amplifiers still leave room for a gain improvement of about 12 dB. But merely increasing the gain causes a restriction of dynamic range by the same amount, thereby limiting the practical usefulness of the aid. In order to improve the overall performance of MEI and widen their scope of application, the gain and maximum output level must both be increased in conjunction. Key factors for achieving this purpose are the vibrator and the battery. If, for example, the vibrator sensitivity could be increased by 10 dB, both gain and maximum output level would be improved by 10 dB, even with all other factors being equal. Taking the half-gain rule into consideration, the practical application range would increase by about 20 dB, making the MEI suitable for patients with a sensorineural hearing impairment from 30 to 50 dB.

Such an increase in vibrator sensitivity will require the development of piezoelectric material with a higher sensitivity, which is by no means an easy task.

On the other hand, if a battery can be developed which provides twice the output voltage and electric capacity at the same size, the maximum output level would be improved by about 6 dB, extending the application scope of the MEI by about 12 dB. However, this also is a goal which will be very hard to realize.

As seen in this light, improving the performance of the T-MEI will be a difficult and slow process. The P-MEI offers a brighter prospect for the future, as improvements in the performance of the external component will be easier to achieve. For example by employing a lithium-manganese oxide battery with higher voltage and electrical capacity, the power of the amplifier in the external component can be boosted, thereby increasing the performance of the inner component by more than 6 dB without making direct alterations to it.

Development of the MEI was concluded only very recently, and at present clinical tests are underway. Engineering reliability must be improved and evaluation methods and standards still need to be set. It is the hope of these authors that the MEI may contribute to the general progress of audiology and hearing aids worldwide.

References

Fukuyama, K.; Yamamoto, T.; Masaike, H.; Suzuki, J.; Kodera, K.: Composition and specification of the implantable hearing aids. Tech. Rep. of the Hearing Research Group, No. H-83-46, pp. 1–8 (Acoustical Society of Japan, Tokyo 1983).

Shono, H.; Takinishi, K.; Ikeda, H.; et al.: The implantable hearing aid. Final Tech. Rep., pp. 90–97 (Technology Research Association of Medical and Welfare Apparatus, Tokyo 1983).

Tohru Ohno, Rion Co., Ltd., Kokubunji Tokyo 185 (Japan)

Experimental Assessment

Adv. Audiol., vol. 4, pp. 97–106 (Karger, Basel 1988)

Evaluation of the Ceramic Vibrator in the Cat

Kazuoki Kodera[a], Hitoshi Yamane[a], Katsumi Suzuki[b], Tohru Ohno[b]

[a] Department of Otolaryngology, Teikyo University School of Medicine, Tokyo;
[b] Rion Co., Ltd., Tokyo, Japan

Introduction

The output transducer is the most important part of a middle ear implant (MEI). The transducer must be as small as possible and implantable in the middle ear; it must perform excellently and have long durability in vivo. Energy consumption must be minimal to qualify the transducer for use as a totally implantable MEI (T-MEI). A piezoelectric ceramic bimorph fulfills the above requirements.

A partially implantable MEI (P-MEI) consists of an output transducer (vibrator) and an internal induction coil. The induction coil can easily be protected by thick biocompatible materials. In any case, the encapsulation of the vibrator should not decrease its performance to any marked degree.

Prior to the clinical application of a P-MEI, animal experiments were carried out to confirm the performance of the vibrator by means of a capacitive probe and by measuring the auditory-evoked brain stem responses (ABRs) [Kodera and Suzuki, 1981]. In the next phase, chronic experiments were performed to confirm the efficacy of the vibrator in vivo for 1 year. The results of these experiments are reported below.

Measurement of the Performance of the Vibrator with the Capacitive Probe

The vibrator used in animal experiments consists of piezoelectric ceramics with a bimorph structure. The vibrator was 7 mm in length, 1 mm in width and 0.4 mm in thickness. One of its tips has a silver wire

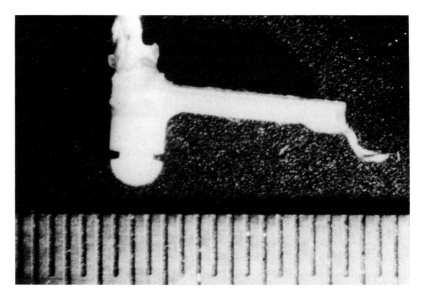

Fig. 1. A photograph of a vibrator consisting of piezoelectric ceramics. The vibrator is 7 mm in length, 1 mm in width and 0.4 mm in thickness. The tip of the vibrator has a silver wire for attachment to the stapes.

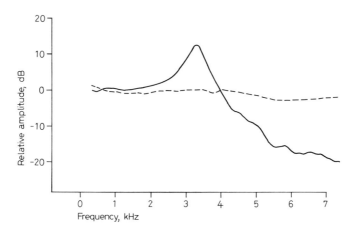

Fig. 2. Frequency responses of the vibrator before and after attachment between the tip and the stapes. After attachment, the resonance at 3,300 Hz disappeared and the sensitivity at 1,000 Hz was preserved.

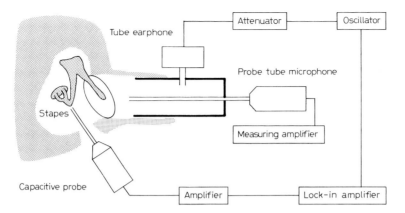

Fig. 3. Block diagram of the measuring system using a capacitive probe. It was used for amplitude measurement of the incudostapedial joint and the vibrator.

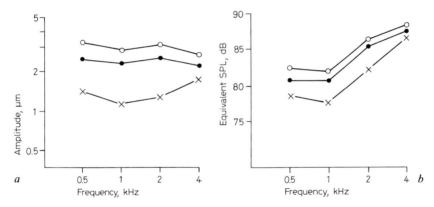

Fig. 4. Amplitudes of the tip of the vibrator attached to the stapes *(a)* in 3 cats, and corresponding SPL, to the amplitudes *(b)*.

for attachment to the stapes, and the other tip has a base made of apatite (fig. 1). The vibrator was coated by PTEF for electrical shielding. Amplitude and frequency responses of the vibrator, measured with a capacitive probe, are shown in figure 2. The resonance frequency of the vibrator was about 3,300 Hz before implantation. After attachment between the tip of the vibrator and the stapes, the resonance disappeared and the sensitivity of the vibrator at 1,000 Hz was preserved.

In a preliminary experiment, the vibration amplitude by air conduction stimuli of the incudostapedial joint was measured in cats as a basis to calculate the performance of the vibrator. A measuring system using the capacitive probe is illustrated in figure 3. The results of the measurement of amplitudes of the incudostapedial joint in 6 cats agreed with the stapes amplitude induced by sound stimuli, as reported by Guinan and Peake [1967].

Using the same device, the amplitudes of the vibrator were measured after implantation in the middle ear in 3 cats. Figure 4 shows the amplitude of the tip of the vibrator attached to the stapes in the middle ear and the values corresponding to sound pressure level (SPL) at the tympanic membrane, calculated from the amplitude of the vibrator. If the connection between the vibrator and the stapes is sufficient, the vibrator can transduce electrical signals to effective vibration in the stapes. The SPLs correspond to 80 dB SPL at 1,000 Hz and 90 dB SPL at 4,000 Hz, when 1 V is charged to the vibrator.

The high fidelity of this vibrator to move the stapes was confirmed in this experiment. Using the same device to evaluate the implanted vibrator, the acoustical wave patterns from the earphone and the vibrations of the incus were measured. The vibrations at the tip of the vibrator with electrical stimuli were similar to the electrical wave patterns. On the other hand, acoustic waves measured in the external auditory canal by probe tube microphone demonstrated distortion, especially at low frequency. Acoustic distortion was noted in the occluded external canal when an earphone was used as hearing aid. The distortion was smaller on the vibration of the incus. It may have been improved at the incus by inertia of the tympanic membrane and the ossicular chains. The results indicate smaller distortion of the vibrator compared to a conventional hearing aid, and higher tonal quality of the MEI.

Measurement of the Efficacy of the Vibrator by ABRs in Cats

Method

Five cats were used in this experiment. All had normal ears as determined by otoscopy and ABRs. Each cat was anesthetized with pentobarbital (38 mg/kg) by intraperitoneal injection. The tympanic membrane was visualized by amputating the pinna; the opposite ear was occluded. The animal was placed in an electrically shielded and sound-attenuated room.

ABRs were recorded from the midline electrode under the skin at the midline of the skull 30 mm anterior to the inion, referenced behind the bulla of the nonstimulated ear; the opposite arm electrode served as a ground connection. First, ABRs evoked by air conduction stimuli were recorded. The stimuli were tone pips with 3 ms rise and decay times at 500, 1,000 and 2,000 Hz, and 1 ms rise and decay times at 4,000 Hz.

Next, surgery was carried out to implant the vibrator to the middle ear in the same cat. The tympanic membrane, malleus and incus were removed and the lateral wall of the attic was opened. The silver wire of the vibrator was attached to the head of the stapes and fixed by dental cement. The base was fixed to the bony wall of the attic by dental cement as well. Again, ABRs to vibration stimuli to the stapes were recorded by applying electrical signals to the vibrator. The waveforms of these electrical signals were the same as those derived by earphone for auditory stimuli. The efficacy of the vibrator was evaluated by comparing the ABRs to the two kinds of stimulus by auditory input and vibration of the stapes.

Results

Recordings of the ABRs to auditory stimuli and vibration stimuli in a cat are shown in figure 5. The recordings to the two kinds of stimulus were very similar to each other at various stimulus intensities. The ABR threshold was 30 dB SPL to the auditory stimuli and −60 dB re 1 V to the vibration stimuli. Calculated from these thresholds, vibration stimuli by charging 1 V to the vibrator correspond to 90 dB SPL at the tympanic membrane. Mean thresholds to auditory and vibration stimuli, obtained from 5 cats, are shown in table I. Output levels of the vibrator by charging 1 V, obtained by calculating the two mean values, are also shown. The output levels correspond well to the values expected from the amplitude measurement by the capacitive probe, as shown in figure 4.

Amplitudes of the ABR to the two kinds of stimulus, measured from vertex-positive peak to the following negative deflection, were obtained at various intensity levels from the 5 cats. Figure 6a shows mean amplitude obtained from the 5 cats. Charging 0 dB re 1 V to the vibrator, as transduced to stapes vibration, corresponds to 90 dB SPL at the tympanic membrane and −50 dB corresponds to 40 dB SPL. Vibration stimuli by charging voltage to the vibrator from 0 dB to −50 dB correspond to sound stimuli from 90 to 40 dB at each of the intensity levels.

Latencies of the ABRs, measured from stimulus onset to the vertex-positive peak, were also obtained from the 5 cats. Figure 6b shows the mean and 1 SD of the latency values at each of the intensity levels of the ABR recordings to two kinds of stimuli. The latencies of the ABRs to vibration stimuli were shorter than those to auditory stimuli by about 0.18 ms at each intensity level. The difference corresponded well to the conduc-

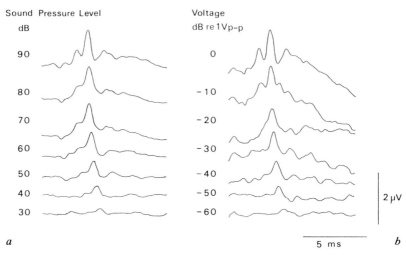

Fig. 5. Recordings of ABRs to auditory *(a)* and vibration *(b)* stimuli in a cat. The recordings to the two kinds of stimulus were very similar to each other at various stimulus intensities. The vibration stimuli by charging 1 V to the vibrator correspond to 90 dB SPL at the tympanic membrane [from Kodera et al., 1981].

Table I. Output of the vibrator by charging 1 V at 500, 1,000, 2,000 and 4,000 Hz obtained from 5 cats

	500 Hz	1,000 Hz	2,000 Hz	4,000 Hz
Threshold to auditory stimuli, dB SPL	43	40	34	35
Threshold to vibration stimuli, dB re 1 V	–32	–39	–51	–55
Calculated output of vibrator, dB SPL/1 V	75	79	85	90

Corresponding SPL at the tympanic membrane was calculated from the stimulus intensities at the response thresholds.

tion time of sound stimuli from the earphone to the stapes. At the vibration stimuli, electrical signals moved the vibrator directly through stapes vibration start faster than sound stimuli. As the difference in latency was identical at each stimulus intensity, this also indicates that vibration stim-

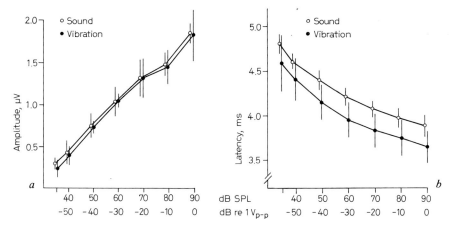

Fig. 6. Mean amplitudes of ABRs to auditory and vibration stimuli from 5 cats *(a)*, and mean latency *(b)*. Charging 0 dB re 1 V to the vibrator, as transduced to stapes vibration, corresponded to 90 dB SPL auditory stimuli. The difference in latency is caused by the conduction time of sound stimuli from the earphone to the stapes.

uli by charging voltage to the vibrator from 0 dB to −50 dB corresponded with sound stimuli from 90 dB to 40 dB at each of the intensity levels.

Experiment to Assess the Efficacy of the Vibrator in vivo for 12 Months

Method

The vibrator used in chronic animal experiments was improved for long-term implantation as compared to that used in acute experiments. It was shortened to 4.5 mm from 7 mm to be completely implantable in the middle ear. At its tip a small apatite was attached instead of a silver wire for contact with the head of the stapes. A connector was installed at the end of the lead wire. The connector was fixed to the vertex of the skull and used to charge voltage to the vibrator.

Surgery was performed to implant the vibrator under anesthesia with pentobarbital (38 mg/kg) by intraperitoneal injection. Incision was made along the pinna and the surface of the temporal bone was explored. The external auditory canal, tympanic membrane, and bony annulus was not injured. The lateral wall of the attic was opened and the malleus head and incus were removed. The apatite tip of the vibrator was attached to the stapes head. The base of the vibrator was fixed near the tegmen of the tympani just above the tendon of the tenor tympani muscle. The upper surface of the vibrator was in contact with subcutaneous tissue near the base, however, most of the vibrator was implanted in the middle ear cavity.

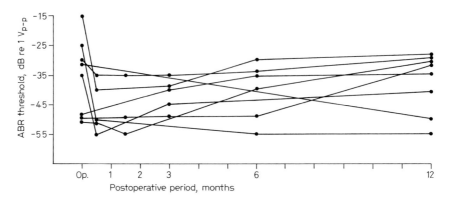

Fig. 7. Results of the long-term follow-up of the vibrator in 8 cats. ABR thresholds to vibration stimuli to the stapes were plotted.

The efficacy of the vibrator was evaluated by repeated ABR measurements during the observation period of 12 months. The method of measurement of ABRs was the same as in the acute experiments.

Results

ABR thresholds at various postoperative periods in 8 cats were shown in figure 7. Just after the operation, the ABR thresholds ranged from −15 to −50 dB re 1 V. At that time, the connection between the tip of the vibrator and the stapes was loose as compared to acute experiments, when dental cement was used to connect them. Two weeks later, the ABR threshold ranged between −35 and −55 dB. Biological reaction fastened the connection between the vibrator and the stapes in 4 cats. Twelve months after the operation, the ABR thresholds ranged from −30 to −55 dB. During the observation periods of 12 months, the performance of the vibrator was maintained. Some cats showed elevation of their ABR thresholds, indicating deterioration in the efficacy of the vibrator, however, the degree of deterioration was fairly small.

Figure 8 demonstrates the connection between the vibrator and the stapes observed by scanning electron microscope. After the observation period of 12 months, the vibrator and stapes were covered and connected by mucous membrane. The membrane was slightly thickened, as observed in human second-look operations in tympanoplasty; however, no active inflammation in the middle ear or deformity of the stapes was observed.

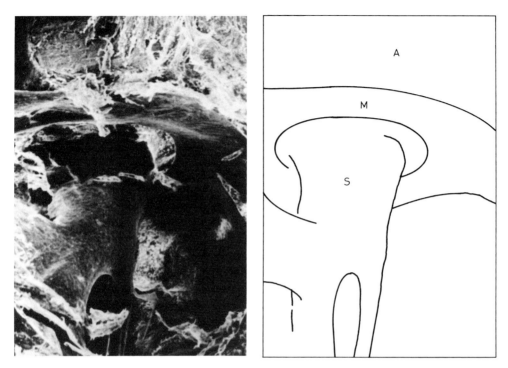

Fig. 8. Scanning electron microradiograph showing the connection between the vibrator and the stapes, 12 months after implantation. Stapes (S), apatite tip (A), mucous membrane over the apatite (M).

Discussion

The vibrator, consisting of piezoelectric ceramics with a bimorph structure, could transduce electrical signals to effective vibration in the stapes. The results of measurements by means of a capacitive probe and ABRs agreed well with each other. ABRs to the vibration and auditory stimuli were very similar to each other at the stimulus intensities in the 50-dB range. The SPLs correspond to 75 dB SPL at 500 Hz, 80 dB SPL at 1,000 Hz, 85 dB SPL at 2,000 Hz and 90 dB SPL at 4,000 Hz when 1 V is charged to the vibrator. The vibrator has satisfactory performance characteristics as a component of the MEI.

Just after the implantation of the vibrator in chronic experiments, ABR threshclds were higher in some cats compared to those in acute experiments. The reason was a loose connection between the tip of the vibrator and the stapes. The connection was fastened by a biological reaction in some cats. In human application of the MEI, the connection would be fastened as in animal experiments. An optimal connection between vibrator and stapes will ensure excellent frequency responses, as reported in this book.

During the observation periods of 12 months, the ability of the vibrator was maintained. Some cats showed deterioration in the efficacy of the vibrator, however, the degree of deterioration was small. The vibrator has excellent performance and durability as a component of the MEI.

Kazuoki Kodera, MD, Department of Otolaryngology,
Teikyo University School of Medicine, Itabashi-ku, Tokyo 173 (Japan)

Adv. Audiol., vol. 4, pp. 107–116 (Karger, Basel 1988)

Measurement of Stapes Vibration Driven by the Ceramic Vibrator of a Middle Ear Implant – Human Temporal Bone Experiments

Kiyofumi Gyo[a], Richard L. Goode[b]

[a] Department of Otolaryngology, Ehime University, School of Medicine, Ehime, Japan; [b] Department of Surgery, Stanford University Medical Center, Stanford, Calif.; Otolaryngology Section, V.A. Medical Center, Palo Alto, Calif., USA

A middle ear implant (MEI), in which a vibrator is directly coupled to the stapes and activates it via an electric signal, has been developed in Japan. This type of MEI is considered to improve the fidelity of sound perception with a minimal consumption of electrical energy. In the development of the MEI, the ossicular vibrator is the most important component. By comparing various types of transducers, a piezoelectric type made of lead zirconate titanate ceramic was selected as the vibrator for the MEI because of its small size, wide frequency range, linear gain and very low distortion and power requirement.

Before actual use in a patient, it was necessary for the functional characteristics of this component to be thoroughly studied. Although engineering tests, animal experiments and clinical tests showed that the physical properties of the vibrator were good enough for practical implantation, the nature of the optimal vibrator-stapes articulation remained unclear. The purpose of the present study was to reveal (1) the vibration mode of the stapes driven by the vibrator, (2) the effect of tight and loose connections on the transmission of vibration, (3) the efficiency of gluing the articulation and (4) the sensitivity of the vibrator when coupled to the head of the stapes.

Materials and Methods

Since the acoustic characteristics of animals are different from those of humans, the following experiments were performed with fresh temporal bones from human cadavers. The specimens were obtained within 24 h of death using a Schuknecht electric saw. They were inspected using a Zeiss operating microscope in order to rule out pathology and then either used immediately or stored in 1:10,000 thimersal (Merthiolate) solution at 5 °C and used within 6 days. In this experiment, 7 temporal bones were used. In order to maintain the acoustic characteristics, the bone samples were kept moist, placed in a rubber finger cot and cemented into a bone holder with dental cement. All cellular openings to the outside were sealed with dental cement.

First, the stapes displacement produced by sound stimuli at the tympanic membrane (TM) was measured. This was performed in order to compare the stapes displacement produced by the vibrator with that produced by normal air conduction in the same temporal bone. Vibrator sensitivity could then be expressed in terms of the equivalent sound pressure level (SPL) at the TM. A 1-mm hole was drilled in the wall of the bony external auditory canal 2–3 mm from the TM, and a Brüel and Kjaer (B & K) model 4170 probe microphone was placed through the hole and hooked up to a microphone amplifier (B & K model 2603). The sound source was a University ID-40 T speaker driver with a rubber tube connected to the external auditory canal via a speculum. The speaker was driven by a B & K model 1027 beat frequency oscillator (BFO) which was synchronized with a B & K stroboscope model 4911. The SPL at the TM was controlled by the probe microphone in the ear canal. Before testing, a thin coat of safflower oil was placed on the TM. Displacement measurements were obtained using the stroboscopic light synchronized to the BFO output and a video measuring system (VMS, Technical Instrument Co.) mounted on a Leitz Laborlux 12 ME microscope. The objective lens used was a Leitz LL 20×/0.40 with a focal distance of 10.1 mm. The viewing axis was through a 4-mm hole drilled in the tegmen that was sealed with a glass cover slip. The bone holder was adjusted to make the stapes approximately perpendicular to the viewing axis. Before sealing the middle ear cavity, stainless steel microspheres 10–60 μm in diameter were placed on the head of the stapes. These reference particles were then observed under stroboscopic illumination at a magnification of × 1,000 using the TV monitor of the VMS, while the microscope was focused on one of the particles on the stapes. The displacement of the particle could be observed in slow motion or stopped at any point along its cyclic path by adjusting the strobe. Peak-to-peak displacement of the stapes was determined by measuring the motion of the reference particle. Measurement of the stapes displacement was performed in response to a constant 124 dB SPL at the TM from 0.1 to 2 kHz. The VMS was calibrated with a stage micrometer and was accurate down to a displacement of 0.3 μm. The details of displacement measurement with the VMS were presented in a previous paper [1987].

After baseline measurement of stapes displacement, the incudostapedial joint was carefully dislocated and the incus, malleus and TM were removed. Then, the vibrating end of the vibrator was positioned on the head of the stapes via a porous polyethylene tip (Plasti-Pore) 1 mm in diameter, 1.5 mm long attached to the end of the vibrator. The long axis of the vibrator element was positioned in approximately the same position as the long process of the incus. The other end was attached to a stainless steel post which was anchored to the bony wall of the middle ear with wax and dental cement (fig. 1). The vibrator was hooked up to the BFO via a B & K model 2606 amplifier and the stimulus voltage was maintained at 100 V_{p-p} at all test frequencies. The stroboscope was synchronized with the frequency of the input to the vibrator in use. Beginning at 0.1 kHz, measurements were made at 0.2-kHz intervals between 0.2 and 3 kHz and at 0.5-kHz intervals between 3 and 8 kHz. Figure 2 shows the set-up of the equipment

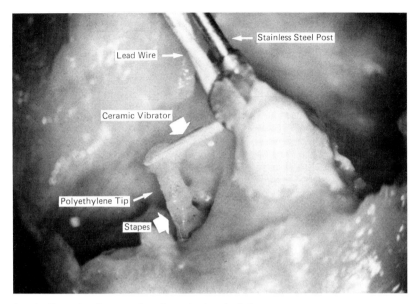

Fig. 1. Ceramic vibrator placed on the head of the stapes.

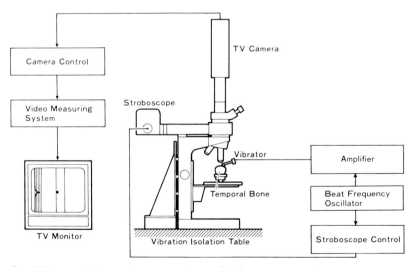

Fig. 2. Set up of the equipment used to make the measurement.

used for measuring the displacements of the vibrator and the stapes. The method of displacement measurement was the same as that mentioned earlier in this section.

The vibrator used in the present study was a piezoelectric ceramic bimorph element which was constructed in the form of a flat chip 5 mm in length, 1.2 mm in width and 0.6 mm in thickness; the element was coated with three different resin layers composed of biocompatible materials. The details of the structural and functional characteristics of the vibrator are described in the earlier sections of this book.

Results

Figure 3 shows the baseline stapes displacement produced by air conduction in normal fresh human temporal bones with the TM and ossicles still in place. The stimulus sound was a constant 124 dB SPL at the TM. The stapes displacement decreased sharply above 1 kHz; measurements were possible up to 2 kHz.

The main advantage of visual measurement is the ability to watch the movement of the vibrator and that of the stapes in slow motion when a stroboscope is used as the light source. The unloaded vibration mode of this piezoelectric element was basically rotatory around an axis located at the nonvibrating end of the vibrator. When the stapes was activated by the vibrator, it vibrated in an arc-like fashion around the same axis (fig. 4). Therefore, the amplitude of the stapes displacement tended to differ with respect to the site on the stapes where the measurement was performed. In subsequent experiments, we used a particle on the midportion of the head of the stapes which was viewed from the tegmen.

There are three general categories of articulation which could be described as 'tight', 'optimal' or 'loose' connections. To make a tight connection, a piece of glass measuring 0.3 mm in thickness was inserted into the joint after the tip had been secured in what was considered to be an optimal connection through microscopic observation. A loose connection was made simply by loosening the anchored post end of the vibrator by manual adjustment. As expected, test-retest reliability was good for a tight connection but poor for a loose connection. Three temporal bones were used for this experiment. Figure 5 shows a typical example of the frequency response curves produced by (1) the vibrator alone, (2) an optimal connection, (3) a tight connection, and (4) a loose connection. These are individual examples of our results; needless to say, there was variation in amplitude between bones, especially with the loose connection. The decrease of displacement due to insertion of the glass was about 3 dB at 1 kHz, although in two other bones in which this procedure was repeated, we found a similar flat response curve with a displacement attenuation of 5 and 10 dB at 1 kHz.

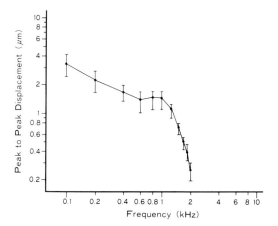

Fig. 3. Average peak-to-peak displacement of the head of the stapes in 7 normal fresh human temporal bones at 124 dB SPL at the tympanic membrane.

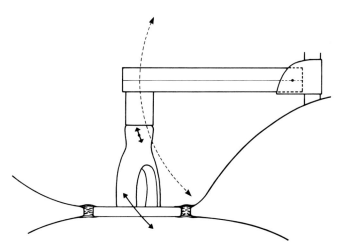

Fig. 4. Vibration mode of the stapes. The stapes vibrates in an arc-like fashion around the same axis of the vibrator.

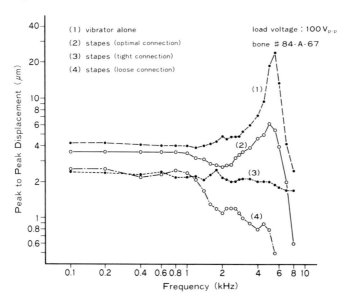

Fig. 5. Peak-to-peak displacements of the vibrator (1) and the stapes activated by the vibrator with three different types of articulation; optimal connection (2), tight connection (3) and loose connection (4).

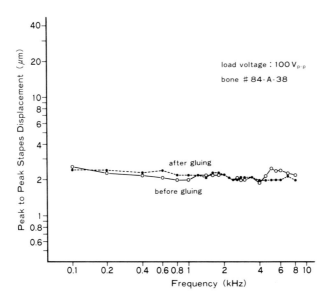

Fig. 6. Effect of gluing a joint with a tight connection. Gluing the joint in this connection had no effect on the frequency response curve.

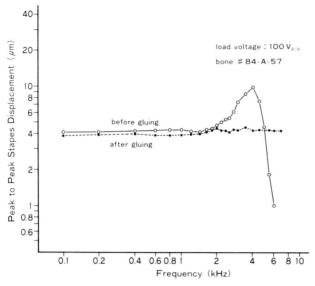

Fig. 7. Effect of gluing a joint with an optimal connection. When the joint was fixed with glue, the frequency response curve became flat and similar to that seen with the tightly loaded connection.

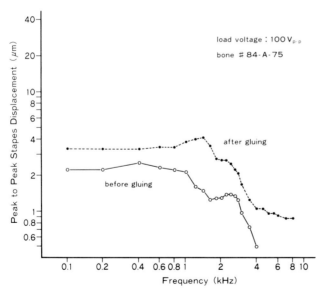

Fig. 8. Effect of gluing a loose connection. Gluing the joint was effective to some extent in improving transmission, but it was unable to maximize the potential of the vibrator especially at high frequencies.

The efficiency of gluing the vibrator to the head of the stapes was studied for the above three conditions using six temporal bones, including two of the bones used for the above experiment. The vibrator tip consisted of a porous polyethylene strut, which in the implant condition would be fixed to the stapes. Therefore, this fixation is important in evaluating the function of the vibrator. In the following experiments, cyanoacrylate glue was used to attach the vibrator to the head of the stapes. Once the joint was glued, it was almost impossible to remove the vibrator from the stapes without damaging the annular ligament of the stapes, so that test-retest reliability could not be assessed in this experiment. The results for two bones in each of the three conditions were consistent, with only minor differences in the degree of changes. Figure 6 shows a typical example when the connection was tight and the joint was glued. In this situation, gluing had no significant effect on the transmission. Figure 7 shows an example of when the connection was optimal and the joint glued. Gluing caused decreased transmission and flattened the frequency response curve. The result was similar to that obtained with insertion of the glass as shown in figure 5. Figure 8 shows an example of a loose connection before and after gluing the connection. Gluing improved the transmission at all frequencies, although, the transmission at higher frequencies was still less than the potential maximum of the vibrator, as determined by measuring the stapes displacement for the same voltage input under tight or optimal conditions.

Discussion

In the present experiment, we used 5-mm-long elements with an unloaded resonance at 5.5 kHz. Our previous experiment using a capacitive probe showed that the longer the element was, the lower the frequency response and the higher the sensitivity. We found that, compared to a 5-mm-long element, a 6-mm-long one had a resonance at 4.5 kHz with a 2-dB increase in sensitivity, whereas a 7-mm-long one had a resonance at 2.5 kHz with a 4-dB increase in sensitivity.

The connection between the vibrator tip and the stapes is critical for obtaining the maximum potential of the vibrator. This situation can be compared with incus substitution in reconstructive surgery of the middle ear in which excessive, optimal and inadequate lengths of the incus substitutes are interposed between the malleus and the head of the stapes.

Elbrond and Elpern [1965] studied this problem using human cadaver temporal bones and showed that excessive length of the substitute caused a reduced sound transmission for low frequencies with a slightly better transmission than the baseline condition at higher frequencies. Conversely, inadequate length caused no loss for low frequencies and substantial loss for high frequencies. Optimal length resulted in transmission closely approximating the baseline condition.

The effect of gluing the connection is also important, because the tip of the vibrator in contact with the stapes will probably become fixed in time in an actual implant. This was simulated by putting glue on the connection. The results showed an increase in transmission only when glue was used on a loose articulation.

Considering the above-mentioned factors, the present results can be interpreted as follows. In the case of a tight connection, the frequency response curve is flat, though the situation is similar to what which occurs when an incus substitute of excessive length is used. This is because in a tight connection the impedance of the stapes and inner ear is loaded on the vibrator, damping its frequency characteristics. As expected, gluing the joint in this connection had no effect. In the case of an optimal connection, the frequency response curve was flat at low frequencies, decreased a little around 2 kHz and showed a peak at 5.5 kHz. This latter peak corresponds to the resonance peak of the unloaded element. The decrease in stapes vibration compared with that of the vibrator alone was small. However, when the joint was fixed with glue, the frequency response curve became flat and similar to that seen with the tightly loaded connection. Therefore, the optimal connection apparently included a degree of looseness. Since the vibrator tip-stapes connection is eventually expected to be fixed as part of the postoperative healing process, the optimal and tight connections may be regarded as the same. In the case of a loose connection, loss of transmission at higher frequencies was prominent. Gluing the joint was effective to some extent in improving transmission, but it was unable to maximize the potential of the vibrator especially at high frequencies. A loose connection should therefore be avoided in actual implantation of the vibrator.

Sensitivity of the vibrator was described in terms of equivalent stapes displacement produced in a normal middle ear by air conduction. Since the stapes displacement at 124 dB SPL was 1.5 μm at 1 kHz and a glued optimal connection at 100 V_{p-p} produced a displacement of 3 μm at 1 kHz in the case of figure 5, we were able to estimate the hearing evoked by the vibrator – vibratory hearing – to be equivalent to 130 dB SPL at the TM. Taking this one step further, because the voltage-to-displacement relationship has been shown to be linear at least between 1 and 100 V_{p-p}, we were also able to estimate that 1 V_{p-p} would be equivalent to 90 dB SPL at the TM. The average sensitivity of the vibrator obtained by this method from 7 temporal bones was represented as 90.9 ± 2.7 dB SPL/1 V_{p-p}, when it was coupled to the head of the stapes at optimal connection. This value is almost identical to that obtained in the clinical tests previously reported.

When the frequency response curve of the stapes displacement activated by the vibrator is flat, as in the case of a tight connection or an optimal glued connection, the threshold curve of the vibratory hearing is expected to be the inverse of the frequency response curve of the stapes displacement by air conduction. Therefore, as the stapes displacement by air conduction decreases sharply above 1 kHz (fig. 3), the vibratory hearing should be improved above 1 kHz. This seems rather beneficial for the design of the amplifier in the MEI, because more amplification is usually necessary at higher frequencies.

The vibration mode of the stapes activated by the vibrator is important in the design and setup of the vibrator. As shown in figure 4, the stapes moves in an arc-like fashion when activated by the vibrator. Such a movement may be less efficient as compared with the usual perpendicular piston-like movement, and might become a problem if a short element or a long tip were to be used. In order to obtain better performance, therefore, the vibrator should be long, the position of the base low, the size of the tip small, and the tip-stapes joint optimal. Gluing the joint will be unnecessary unless the joint is loose.

References

Gyo, K.; Aritomo, H.; Goode, R. L.: Measurement of the ossicular vibration ratio in human temporal bones by use of a video measuring system. Acta oto-lar. *103:* 87–95 (1987).

Elbrond, O.; Elpern, B. S.: Reconstruction of ossicular chain in incus defects. An experimental study. Arch. Otolar. *82:* 603–608 (1965).

K. Gyo, MD, Department of Otolaryngology, Ehime University
School of Medicine, Shigenobu-cho, Onsen-gun, Ehime 791-02 (Japan)

Adv. Audiol., vol. 4, pp. 117–123 (Karger, Basel 1988)

Evaluation of the Implantable Microphone in the Cat

Kazuoki Kodera[a], Katsumi Suzuki[b], Tohru Ohno[b]

[a] Department of Otolaryngology, Teikyo University School of Medicine, Tokyo;
[b] Rion Co., Ltd., Tokyo, Japan

Introduction

An implantable microphone is an indispensable part of a totally implantable middle ear implant (T-MEI). Of course, this microphone must be placed just under the skin adjacent to the ear. The ideal site of implantation is the external auditory canal, where the resonance of the pinna and the external auditory canal can be utilized. Thus, the microphone has to be small enough. It also must have excellent performance characteristics and durability in vivo for a long period.

Keeping these requirements in mind, an electret microphone was developed and tested [Kodera and Suzuki, 1981; Araki et al., 1983]. Another microphone, a ceramic type, which is more durable and water-resistant, has also been considered. Still, the electret microphone, if it can be made water-resistant, seems the best choice. Its electroacoustic performance is excellent and it can easily be miniaturized.

Two major questions remain before a successful implantable microphone can be fully perfected: To what extent is its efficacy decreased when implanted under the skin? Is it possible to insulate the microphone while preserving its performance? This paper reports the progress of experiments carried out to provide answers to these questions. The results of a chronic experiment involving a T-MEI are given as well.

Structure and Performance of the Implantable Microphone

The structure of the implanted microphone is described in another chapter of this book. An electret microphone unit converting sounds into voltages is encased in stainless steel. The front surface of the case consists of a 9-μm-thick stainless steel diaphragm through which sounds enter the microphone. The air space surrounding the microphone unit is filled with argon gas, so as to protect the mechanism from tissue fluid. A hermetic terminal is used to separate the microphone from the outside and epoxy thoroughly coats the silver lead wire to protect it from tissue fluid as well. The purpose of the lead wire is twofold: to measure the efficacy of the microphone and to supply energy.

The sensitivity of the implantable microphone in the free field is −55 dB (0 dB = 1 V/μbar), the frequency response is flat from 500 to 4,000 Hz and the resonance frequency is about 10,000 Hz, resulting from a 9-μm-thick diaphragm (fig. 1).

Animal Experiments

Five cats were used in this experiment. They were anesthetized with pentobarbital (38 mg/kg, intraperitoneal injection). The skin was incised above the skull from the line of the left pinna to the right orbital margin. The skin of the vertex was then reflected and the microphone fixed to the occipital bone by screws and the lead wire fixed apart. The connector was not used at the other terminal of the lead wire. This precaution was taken since, in a preliminary attempt to evaluate the implantable microphone, a connector had caused a skin infection that had decreased the performance of the implanted microphone [Suzuki et al., 1983]. A collar was used to protect the microphone from damage by contact between the cat's head and the cage.

During the 6 months of testing, the sensitivity of the microphone was checked repeatedly. Sounds were applied and their output voltage was measured. The sound pressure levels (SPLs) at the surface of the skin adjacent to the implanted microphone was monitored by a probe tube microphone.

Results

Figure 1 shows the frequency response of a microphone just after and before implantation in a cat. The resonance frequency changed from 10,000 to 4,000 Hz, this change was caused by the covering skin. The sensitivity of the microphone at 1,000 Hz showed a small decrement; the mean value of this decrement in the 5 cats was only 2 dB (1 SD = 1 dB).

Figure 2 shows the changes of the frequency responses obtained in a cat during a 6-month period. The resonance frequency altered between 3,000 and 5,000 Hz because of a change in skin thickness after the opera-

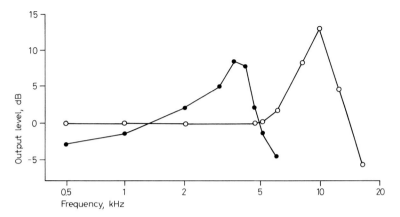

Fig. 1. The frequency response of a microphone just after (●) and before implantation (○) in a cat. The resonance frequency changed from 10,000 to 4,000 Hz after implantation.

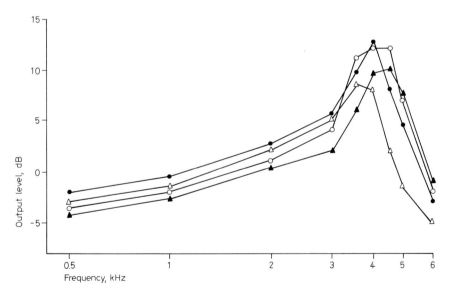

Fig. 2. Changes in the frequency responses of an implanted microphone during a 6-month period. The resonance frequency altered between 3,000 and 5,000 Hz. △ = just after operation; ○ = 6 weeks after; ▲ = 3 months after; ● = 6 months after.

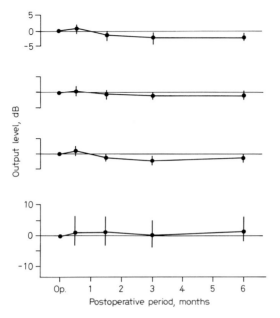

Fig. 3. Mean sensitivity changes of 5 implanted microphones. Vertical bars indicate ranges obtained from 5 cats. The sensitivity was very stable at all frequencies.

tion. The performance of the microphone remained stable during the observation period.

Figure 3 shows the mean sensitivity changes of the implanted microphones at 500, 1,000, 2,000 and 4,000 Hz during the observation period.
The sensitivity was very stable from 500 to 2,000 Hz. The sensitivity at
4,000 Hz showed a relatively large difference which paralleled the change
in resonance frequency.

Efficacy of the Microphone Implanted in the Human External Auditory Canal in the Postoperative State

The sensitivity and frequency response of an implanted microphone
will be altered by the thickness of the covering skin. The thicker the skin,
the lower the resonance frequency. The sensitivity and frequency response was measured in patients undergoing a second-look operation,
because subjects with middle ear disease will receive a T-MEI only after
the first-stage operation.

The external auditory canal, near the tympanic membrane, is an
ideal site for implantation. Open ear gain, by the resonance of the auricle

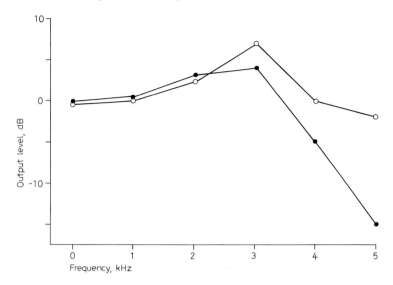

Fig. 4. Frequency response of microphones implanted in the external auditory canals of 2 patients.

and the external auditory canal, can be used. Breakage by accidental external force can be avoided effectively. The implantable microphone was placed beneath the skin of the external canal near the antrum, and a control microphone was set at the external auditory canal, at a distance of 5 mm from the microphone. The sensitivity and frequency response of the microphone was obtained by comparing the outputs of the two microphones. Figure 4 shows the frequency response of the implanted microphone. Resonance frequency is about 3,000 Hz and sensitivity at 1,000 Hz showed no decrement.

Nine-Month Observation of the T-MEI in Cats

Figure 5 shows a photograph of the T-MEI used in our animal experiment. It consists of a microphone, an amplifier, a switch, a vibrator and a battery. The electrical supply was switched on by magnetic force at test, since the size of the battery needed for a cat is too small for continued use. T-MEI implantation was carried out under anesthesia. To implant the vibrator, the lateral wall of the attic was opened and the malleus head and incus were removed. The apatite tip of the vibrator was at-

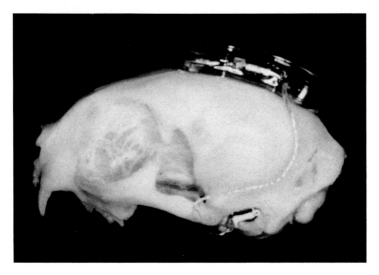

Fig. 5. Photograph of a T-MEI used in animal experiments. It consists of a microphone, an amplifier, a switch, a vibrator and a battery.

tached to the head of the stapes and the base of the vibrator was fixed to the tegmen of the attic with dental cement. The tympanic membrane and the external auditory canal were not injured. Another component of the T-MEI was situated on the vertex under the skin and fixed by dental cement after the vibrator was implanted.

Auditory brain stem responses (ABR) under anesthesia were used to assess the performance of the T-MEI. The ABRs were recorded through a needle electrode under the skin at the midline of the forehead, referenced behind the bulla of the nonstimulated ear. The opposite arm electrode served as a ground connection. To estimate the efficacy of this T-MEI, a switch was turned on with a magnet. Tone pips with 1-ms rise-decay times at 4,000 Hz were sent into the microphone through the skin as auditory stimuli. In order to avoid sound stimulation through the ear, both ears were occluded with clay. If the T-MEI was turned off and both ears remained occluded, the ABR threshold of a cat was 70 dB SPL.

Figure 6 shows the results of the long-term follow-up of a functioning T-MEI, preserved in a cat for 9 months. The ABR threshold to stimulation through the T-MEI increased during the observation period. This deterioration of the T-MEI was mainly caused by two things: the decreased performance of the microphone and the decrement of effective

SPL/V_{p-p} and 2 kHz 100 dB SPL/V_{p-p}. The result indicated that the vibrator had sufficient efficiency for practical use of the MEI.

The group of investigators of Rion Company theoretically estimated the sensitivity of the vibrator of 7 mm length based on an experiment similar to that of Guinan and Peak [1967] using ABR of a cat and on the relationship between oscillation amplitude of the umbo of the eardrum and the stapes in man. The estimated sensitivity is almost the same as that measured at 0.5, 1.0 and 2.0 kHz, as is shown in figure 5. The large discrepancy at 4 kHz may have been caused by a loose connection between the stapes and the tip of the vibrator. Gyo et al. [in press] measured the sensitivity of the same vibrator attached to the stapes of fresh human temporal bone and found the sensitivity of the vibrator to be 91 dB at 1 kHz. These results indicate that the intraoperative measurement of the vibratory hearing threshold and the estimation of the sensitivity we developed are reliable and useful from both the technological and the clinical viewpoints.

Intraoperative Assessment of Hearing Afforded by Partially Implantable MEI.

As described in the previous chapter, we have developed MEI of two types, totally implantable MEI (T-MEI) and partially implantable MEI (P-MEI).

In view of the life of the device, its adjustability to individual peculiarities of patients' hearing and considering the simplicity of the surgical procedure involved, we decided to apply the P-MEI preferentially to selected patients. For this clinical purpose, we needed to develop a method of assessing hearing afforded by the P-MEI before and after the implantation. By preliminary experiments, several theoretically possible methods were examined on the basis of the functional principle of the P-MEI shown in figure 6. We found the following two methods clinically useful.

In the first method, the hearing level afforded by the P-MEI can be estimated from the data of the sensitivity of the vibrator and the transmission gain of the P-MEI. Estimated hearing level afforded by the P-MEI can be obtained by the equation:

estimated hearing level = bone-conduction level – transmission gain – (measured sensitivity – standard sensitivity).

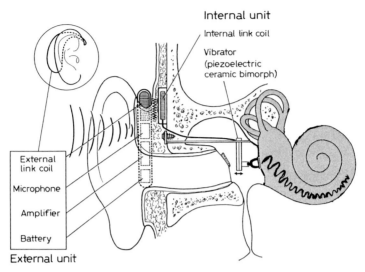

Fig. 6. Functional principle of the P-MEI.

Table I. Standard sensitivity of the vibrator of 7 mm in length and transmission gain of the P-MEI of N type

Frequency Hz	Standard sensitivity dB SPL/1 V_{p-p}	Transmission gain dB
250	84	−11
500	84	− 2
1,000	89	+ 4
2,000	98	+10
4,000	104	+21
6,000	105	+ 5

The standard sensitivity and transmission gain at each test frequency are given in table I.

In the second method, the hearing threshold afforded by the P-MEI can be assessed directly using the internal coil and the outer unit. As shown in figure 7, output signals of the audiometer are fed into the outer testing unit in which the attenuator is incorporated instead of the microphone. The amount of the attenuation is adjusted so that the read decibel value of the audiometer at the vibratory hearing threshold gives the hearing level at 1.0 kHz afforded by the P-MEI. At the other test frequencies,

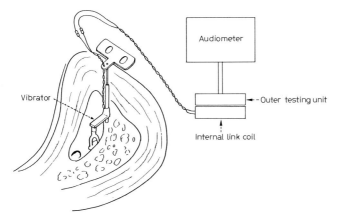

Fig. 7. System of intraoperative assessment of hearing afforded by a P-MEI.

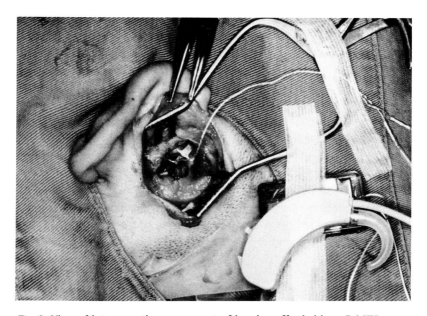

Fig. 8. View of intraoperative assessment of hearing afforded by a P-MEI.

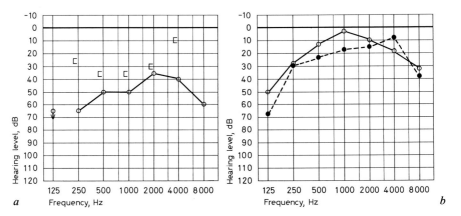

Fig. 9. Representative result of intraoperative test of hearing afforded by a P-MEI. *a* Preoperative audiogram. *b* Hearing level afforded by a P-MEI. --- = Estimated; —— = after implantation.

minor correction of the read decibel value is needed to determine the hearing level. The lead wires of the vibrator were connected to those of the internal coil. The coil in the outer testing unit was placed just above the internal coil that transmits the signals from the audiometer to the vibrator. Figure 8 shows the actual appearance of this intraoperative test.

In the 34 patients, the hearing level afforded by the P-MEI was estimated by the first method and then it was assessed by the second method. In all subjects, no significant discrepancy was noted between the estimated and the assessed hearing level which in turn indicated the high reliability of the methods employed.

After surgical implantation of the internal units of the P-MEI, the vibratory hearing level can be assessed by placing the outer unit on the retroauricular skin covering the internal coil. In figure 9, the hearing levels estimated and assessed during operation and measured after the operation are shown in the form of an audiogram and compared with the preoperative pure-tone audiogram.

We have proved that significant restoration of hearing levels at speech frequencies can be achieved by the P-MEI. As long as the bone-conduction level remains within 30 dB in average at speech frequencies, hearing levels better than 20 dB can be restored. The patient could hear through the P-MEI when the outer unit of the P-MEI was placed on the internal coil instead of the outer testing unit. All the patients recognized that sound quality perceived through the device was clear, pleasant to hear and intelligible. The results of the intraoperative test of the vibratory hearing were verified by implanting the P-MEI into human subjects, as described in a separate chapter.

References

Guinan, J.J., Jr.; Peak, W.T.: Middle ear characteristics of anesthetized cats. J. acoust. Soc. Am. *41:* 1237–1261 (1967).
Gyo, K.; Goode, R.L.; Miller, G.: Experimental study of stapes vibration produced by the output transducer of an implantable hearing aid. Archs Otolar. (in press).
Shaw, E.: Transformation of sound pressure from the free field to the eardrum in the horizontal plane. J. acoust. Soc. Am. *56:* 1848–1861 (1974).

Naoaki Yanagihara, MD, Department of Otolaryngology, Ehime University School of Medicine, Shigenobu-cho, Onsen-gun, Ehime 791–02 (Japan)

Adv. Audiol., vol. 4, pp. 134–148 (Karger, Basel 1988)

Audiological Evaluation of the Middle Ear Implant

Shizuo Hiki[a], Nobuo Takahashi[b]

[a] School of Human Sciences, Waseda University, Tokorozawa;
[b] Faculty of Education, Ehime University, Matsuyama, Japan

In this chapter, the implantation of the artificial middle ear will be reviewed from the viewpoint of audiological evaluation, referring to the data on technical aspects described in part II and on experimental assessment in part III.

The term 'artificial middle ear' is used in this chapter, analogous to 'artificial inner ear', to imply an artificial hearing organ, i.e. an implanted auditory prosthesis. So, it may be called 'middle ear implant' (MEI), in parallel with 'cochlear implant', which is already widely used. But, an electronic auditory prosthesis consisting of a microphone-amplifier-vibrator, comparable to the microphone-amplifier-electrode of the artificial inner ear, is implanted in the artificial middle ear, not as in eardrum implantation, where a part of human tissue is implanted, nor as in ossicular reconstructive surgery, where simple artificial parts are inserted.

The terms 'artificial middle ear', as well as 'artificial inner ear', could be used to express the total concept such as artificial hearing, artificial ear and electronic ear, but 'artificial middle ear' is more often used here for the artificial hearing organ itself. It can be regarded as 'an implantable hearing aid', but the method of transmitting acoustical information is different from the ordinary hearing aids which transmit the vibration of the sound to the eardrum through air conduction or to the inner ear through bone conduction. Sound vibration is converted into an electrical signal and stimulates the inner ear or the auditory nerves directly through the electrode in the artificial inner ear, while in the artificial middle ear, it is converted into a mechanical signal and stimulates the middle ear or the ossicles directly using the vibrator. In order to differentiate the mode of hearing, the sensation induced by the vibrator will be referred to as 'mechanical hearing', in contrast with 'electrical hearing' by the former and 'ordinary hearing' through air and bone conduction.

The discussion in this chapter is based on the experiments conducted at the Department of Otolaryngology, Faculty of Medicine, Ehime University with the partially implantable type of artificial middle ear, in which the microphone, amplifier, primary link coil and battery are placed outside the patient's body, and only the secondary link coil and vibrator are implanted.

Prediction of the Transmission Ability of Sound Information by Mechanical Stimulation of the Middle Ear

The methods and results of the various measurements on mechanical hearing have already been described in detail in the previous chapter of this part. Construction and specification of the artificial middle ear have also been described in parts II and III. In this section, some aspects of audiological evaluation of the MEI will be discussed.

The first topic concerns the analogy of the accuracy of prescriptive fitting of the ordinary hearing aid to the artificial middle ear, the second concerns the experiment on judgements of loudness and tonal quality during tympanoplasty, and the third concerns the selection of speech materials of audiometric tests for the fitting of the artificial middle ear.

Accuracy of Prescriptive Fitting of the Artificial Middle Ear

In the case of ordinary hearing in which vibration of sound in the air is transmitted through the mechanisms of the outer and middle ears, the following items underlie the prescriptive fitting of air-conduction-type hearing aids to conductive and/or sensorineural hearing-impaired patient, and also the prediction of the possibility of transmission of sound information by the aided characteristics. The items are: variations in the amplitude-frequency range of objective sound; accuracy of the measurements of the minimal audible threshold, uncomfortable level and most comfortable level in pure-tone audiometry; correction for the electro-acoustical measurement of the characteristics of the hearing aid required by the actual using condition and the individuality of the user, and especially for the transmission of speech information, dependency of speech audiometry on the phonetic and acoustical properties of the test materials, linguistic and psychological factors such as stage of language development, dialectal and personal accents, and capability for the perceptual test.

In spite of the fact that some errors are possibly introduced by the factors involved in each item, prescriptive fitting of the hearing aid is done at a level of accuracy which leaves little allowable readjustment for the user, when the aided characteristics are predicted from the characteristics of the hearing loss and the hearing aid [Pascoe, 1980]. This prediction can be improved further if all the quantitative data of these factors are combined.

Even in the case of mechanical hearing with the artificial middle ear, in which sound vibration is converted electroacoustically into a mechanical signal and transmitted directly to the inner ear, the previously mentioned factors, except the factor related to the electroacoustical measurement of the hearing aid, are the same as for ordinary hearing.

The factors specific to mechanical hearing described below are related to the physical characteristics of sound transmission by mechanical driving of the middle ear and those of the artificial middle ear including the microphone, amplifier and vibrator.

In order to estimate the transmission characteristics of mechanical hearing, the transmission characteristics from the eardrum to the base of the stapes should be eliminated from the overall transmission characteristics of ordinary hearing, and the resonance characteristics from the inlet of the outer ear to the eardrum should also be eliminated when the microphone is installed outside the body. These estimations can be made based on measured data of those characteristics.

Among the characteristics of the devices, the deterioration of the sensitivity of the electret condenser microphone due to implantation under the skin surface has been observed to be less than 3 dB for −78 dB at 1 kHz in animal experiments. Using the accelerated aging test, the deterioration was also estimated to be less than 6 dB after 4.5 years. According to measurements with the capacitive probe, the variation in the absolute sensitivity of the piezoelectric ceramic type vibrator is about 0.025 μm/V_{p-p} when the mechanical impedance of the inner ear is loaded, whereas according to animal experiments, the decrease in sensitivity is less than 10 dB, except for the initial instability.

In order to avoid the effect of the initial instability immediately after implantation, the overall characteristics, including the circuitry, can be readjusted based on the measurement after stabilization.

The characteristics of the circuitry and battery can be set much more accurately than those of the microphone and the vibrator.

By combining the characteristics of transmission and those of the mechanical hearing devices with the psychoacoustical characteristics of sound perception in the ordinary hearing of hearing-impaired patients, it is possible to predict the aided frequency-amplitude response by mechanical hearing. Consequently, it is possible to predict how the patients perceive the acoustical properties necessary to transmit the various aspects of sound information.

Experiment on Judgements of Loudness and Tonal Quality

As reported in the previous chapter, the sensitivity of the vibrator is ascertained by measuring the minimal audible pure-tone and masking thresholds obtained by mechanical hearing, i.e. by attaching the vibrator to the ossicles during tympanoplasty. Taking into account the variation of attenuation caused by attachment, the sensitivity was within the range predicted by the characteristics of the vibrator itself, which corresponds to about 85 dB SPL at 1 kHz with 1 V_{p-p} input voltage when converted into sound pressure at the eardrum.

It was also ascertained by measurement using masking noise that the linearity was reasonably good. The uncomfortable level was more than 50 dB above the minimal audible threshold and the most comfortable level was at a level in between them.

For patients who could use their better ear during tympanoplasty, the reference tone was delivered through the minireceiver simultaneously with the test tone, which was delivered through the vibrator to the impaired ear. For adjustment of the hearing level in each ear, the patient was requested to judge whether the loudness of the tone heard by the impaired ear was higher than that on the other side or not. A steady pure tone of 1 kHz was used for the test and reference tones.

As a result, the loudness could be matched with a reproducibility of 5 dB to within 10 dB of the condition predicted by the minimal audible threshold. This implies, at the same time, that the sensation of loudness caused by mechanical hearing is not different from that caused by ordinary hearing.

Then, by using a time varying complex tone for the test and reference tone, the frequency responses were adjusted through the equalizers, emphasizing or de-emphasizing the high-frequency components, and successively presented to the impaired ear and the better ear. The patient was asked to judge the difference in tonal quality with reference to a perceptual scale which may be described as sharp versus dull, and to say whether the tonal quality on the impaired side was sharper than on the other side or not.

For the test and reference tones, samples whose frequency spectra and transient properties were suitable for analysis were chosen from sound sources encountered in daily life. They included an indoor speech sound (a weather forecast on the radio broadcast by a male voice), an outdoor speech sound (an announcement at a railway station by a male voice), indoor signal sounds (a telephone ringing and a doorbell), outdoor alarm sounds (the siren of an ambulance car and the horn of a car), musical instruments (a zither and a violin), and sounds in nature (a song of a bird and the tide). All the samples contained ample components at the frequency range up to 5 kHz.

As a result, the difference in tonal quality could be matched to within ±3 dB/oct of the condition predicted by the frequency response of the minimal audible thresholds of the two ears. The frequency range was up to the highest limit of about 5 kHz which was determined by the characteristics of the vibrator. This, again, implies that tonal quality perceived by mechanical hearing was similar to that perceived by ordinary hearing.

If corrections are made for the error in the measurement of the minimal audible pure-tone threshold, the approximation in the adjustment of the frequency response of the equalizer, the difficulty of the patients in responding during the operation, and the discrepancy in the perceptual scale, then, the difference between the predicted value and the observed value can be explained more precisely.

Selection of Speech Materials for Audiometric Tests

The articulation score was examined using lists of Japanese monosyllables which had been arranged especially for this particular test in order to reduce the necessary time and to improve the accuracy.

In contrast to the various speech units used in audiometric tests in English [Levitt, 1980], 100 Japanese monosyllables consisting of preceding consonant and following vowel or semi-vowel, are used as the most basic units of speech in Japanese.

When it is possible to repeat many times the speech intelligibility test with a large number of monosyllables, the optimal figure indicating the patient's hearing ability may be derived directly by considering the probability of the occurrence of each kind of syllable in daily life. However, when only a limited time is allowed for the test as in the case of the test during the operation, it is necessary to use a small number of syllables containing a variety of acoustical features, and estimate the ability of transmission of speech information based on the detailed analysis of the data obtained. The lists of monosyllables arranged for this purpose are as follows:

List of 20 Monosyllables with Unvoiced Consonants. The following 20 monosyllables with unvoiced consonants followed by the 5 Japanese vowels were selected from the speech samples of the 50 monosyllables of list 57 of the Standard Lists for Speech Audiometry established by the Japan Audiological Society and used in all clinics in Japan: [ta, tʃi, tsu, te, to, sa, ʃi, su, se, so, ka, ki, ku, ke, ko, ha, çi, ɸu, he, ho]; they were rearranged and recorded with equal sound levels and intervals. The number of syllables is the same as in list 67 and each vowel appears with the same probability in this list.

List of 20 Monosyllables with Vowels [a] and [i]. They consist of unvoiced and voiced consonants followed by vowel [a]: [ta, sa, ka, ha, ba, da, ga, wa, ja, pa, ma, na] and of the palatalized consonants which appear when followed by vowel [i]: [tʃi, ʃi, ki, çi, dʒi, ri, mi, ni]. They were also selected from the speech samples of list 57.

List of 16 Monosyllables of Unvoiced and Voiced Consonants followed by Vowel [a]. This list is used when the vowel articulation score is high enough but a quick test of the discrimination of consonants is needed. The syllables are: [pa, ta, tʃa, ʃa, ka, ha, ça, ba, da, dza, dʒa, ga, ra, ma, na]. Speech samples were recorded by a speaker having similar acoustical features as the speaker of the Standard List of Speech Audiometry, and the sound level, interval and articulation were carefully controlled.

Using these lists of monosyllables, an articulation score of 100% was obtained at 30 dB above the minimal audible threshold, as was the case for ordinary hearing. The discrimination ability of phones predicted by the aided characteristics was ascertained by analyzing the nature of the confusion among the phones.

The intelligibility of words and sentences can be basically estimated by analyzing the results of the test with the monosyllables, but, by selecting suitable speech materials based on the relationship between the frequency response of the artificial middle ear and the spectral properties of consonants, the discrimination ability of the phones was ascertained with higher accuracy.

The list of the speech materials consists of 25 Japanese words such as: [ʃiho:, onʃi, senʃa, ʃo:ʒo, ʃu:zi, konʃu:] which were selected for a probable confusion of [ʃ→tʃ] caused inevitably by the lack of the frequency components in the range around 4 kHz. [tsu:kai, dentsu:] for [ts→tʃ], [sain, so:ʒi, kanso:, tʃu:su:] for [s→ʃ]. denðaku, daiku, sando:] for [d→b], and [tentʃi, kantan] for [t→p]. All the words have meaningful counterparts for which they can be easily mistaken should the phones be confused.

As reported in the previous chapter, it was also ascertained from the conversation between the operators and the patient that the transmission characteristics were good enough to recognize speech sound as expected from the results of audiometric tests with the pure tones and monosyllables and words, and, in addition, to identify the speakers through differences in the tonal quality of their speech.

Summing up these results of the experiments on judging loudness, tonal quality and speech discrimination, it can be said that the prescriptive fitting of the artificial middle ear for implantation into patients with conductive and/or sensorineural hearing loss is possible with the same accuracy as for ordinary hearing. This requires that the hearing loss characteristics of ordinary hearing and the transmission characteristics of vibratory hearing including the devices, be combined, and some adjustment to the prediction be made based on the measurement of the minimal audible pure-tone threshold during the implantation operation.

Analysis of the Improvement of the Hearing Ability after Implantation of the Artificial Middle Ear

In this section, the improvement of the hearing ability after implantation is analyzed with reference to the discussion on the prediction of the transmission ability of sound information by mechanical stimulation of the middle ear in the previous section. An integrated evaluation of the hearing ability for various sound sources, in addition to pure-tone audiometry and standard speech audiometry, has been conducted on the 5 patients in whom a partially implantable type artificial middle ear was implanted at the Department of Otolaryngology, Faculty of Medicine, Ehime University, in August 1984.

Parameters Assessed

The following measurements were made: minimal audible threshold and the audible amplitude-frequency range (dynamic range), discrimination of tonal quality and the speech intelligibility. The measurements and tests were performed in a sound-proof room in the hospital before and after the operation. All the 5 patients are using the MEI successfully in their daily life. In the following paragraphs, the results of the evaluation of the hearing ability for the various sound sources will be described in detail taking one of the patients as a typical example.

Status of the Hearing Ability of the Patient before the Implantation

The patient is a male aged 61 who has been working in the local government office until 2 years ago when he retired. He has been suffering from hearing disorders in both ears since his childhood, and had a middle ear reconstruction operation in the left ear. As the right ear had few chances of being improved by surgery, it was chosen for the implantation. The hearing levels were 45 dB HL (ANSI, 1969) for the left ear and 56 dB HL for the right. The hearing aids had not been used regularly because he had difficulty in discriminating speech even when using them and had been disturbed by the amplification noise.

In his daily life before the implantation, he could hear a loud alarm sound such as a buzzer, he watched television with a louder sound volume, and the conversation with his wife was understandable as her speech had a higher intensity level. In the conversation with the tester, the patient often misunderstood the instructions, or he had to ask him to repeat and use lipreading, especially when the subject of conversation was changed. He had a good perception of his own speech.

Improvement in the Minimal Audible Threshold and
Audible Range of Amplitude-Frequency Range

The minimal audible threshold was improved from the average hearing level of 55 dB HL before operation to 35 dB HL immediately after the implantation in August 1984, and to 25 dB HL with the artificial middle ear after 1 year. The amount of improvement of the threshold was more than 30 dB above 500 Hz. The values of the threshold for all frequencies approximately correspond to those predicted based on the measurement before operation. They are close to the bone-conduction threshold below 500 Hz and even smaller than that in the high-frequency range above 1 kHz. The variation of the average hearing level during the first week was within only ± 10 dB. The threshold could be decreased further if the volume dial of the amplifier worn outside the body was tuned to the maximum, but, in order to avoid a disturbing noise, it was set at a comfortable level for normal conversation. The threshold was stable even 1 year after the operation, showing the minimum value in the range of variation during the first week after the operation. The value also corresponds to the aided characteristics achieved by the optimum fitting of an ordinary hearing aid.

The audible amplitude-frequency range, estimated by the difference between the minimal audible threshold and the uncomfortable level, which was measured with the noise band around center frequencies of 500 Hz, 1 and 2 kHz, was extended from about 35 dB before the operation to nearly 60 dB with the artificial middle ear. This was not affected by the maximum output level of the amplifier. As the dynamic range of more than 50 dB is difficult to achieve using ordinary hearing aids, this wide dynamic range is considered to be one of the most important advantages of the artificial middle ear.

Discrimination of Tonal Quality

A test for detecting the difference of tonal quality was conducted using the sound of a doorbell with or without high frequency cut-off. The sound was chosen as an example of an indoor signal sound familiar to the patient in order to help him to detect any difference in tonal quality. The duration of the sound was about 5 s and a pair of samples was presented successively with an interval of 2 s between them, and the patient was asked to answer whether they were same or different in their tonal quality. Before the operation, it was impossible to detect any difference between the pair even with a cut-off frequency of up to 1,200 Hz, while with the artificial middle ear, the difference became perfectly detectable at as low as 3,400 Hz. When the high-frequency components were cut off, the patient described the sound as follows: 'The tonal quality became soft and dull.'

The chirping of a grasshopper, as an example of the natural sound, was difficult to perceive before the operation, but it became audible at an intensity level of 50 dB SPL with the MEI. The subjective impression of the tonal quality of various sound sources was expressed by the patient as 'clear (crisp) and natural' for the artificial middle ear versus 'unnatural (strained)' for the ordinary hearing aid which he had been using.

Speech Intelligibility

Before the operation, the articulation score at a sound level of 60 dB was 90% for vowels, most of the errors being found with the vowel [e] and 45% for consonants. The tendency of confusion was found to be similar to that of normal listeners at this low sound level, that is, more confusion for fricatives and affricates having high-frequency components. On the other hand, the articulation score became almost 100% for both vowels and consonants when the MEI was in working condition. This high score was chieved at a sound level of 80 dB before the implantation.

In order to detect the improvement more accurately, a list of 25 words requiring high-frequency components for their identification, which are supposed to become audible with the aided characteristics, was used. A correct response was obtained in about 40% at a sound level of 60 dB before the operation, demonstrating confusions between unvoiced, voiced and nasal consonants and confusions related to the Japanese [r] sound and palatal consonants versus their nonpalatal counterparts. There were less than 50% correct responses with ordinary hearing aids, while the correct responses increased to 90% with the artificial middle ear, leaving few errors in the syllables with semi-vowels. The nature of the error was taken into account in the program of training of hearing ability.

While conducting the above measurements and tests on the hearing ability of patients with the MEI, the methods were reexamined from the viewpoint of the analysis of the data obtained. Some of the points to be revised in the methods are as follows: although it is necessary to check the performance of the artificial middle ear in the sound field, a direct input of the electrical signal through a dummy microphone for the outside-of-the-body unit can be used for a precise measurement if both measurements are calibrated accurately.

In order to secure a stable linkage between the outside- and the inside-of-the-body units through the primary and secondary coils during the whole series of the measurements and tests, special care should be taken with patients who wear eyeglasses.

As a limited time is allowed for the measurements and tests during implantation surgery, the following must be taken into account to obtain as much useful information from the patient as possible; (a) to design the tasks so that the patient can answer with phrases which are simple and easy to pronounce; (b) to select the sounds which are most often encountered in the patient's daily life; (c) to avoid words which were uttered with an accent not common in the patient's dialect, and (d) to train the patient in the tasks under simulated conditions before the operation.

Testing and Training Program for the Recovery of Hearing Ability with the MEI

In this part, the testing and training program for the recovery of hearing is summarized in a general form, based on the predicted ability of the mechanically stimulated middle ear to transmit sound information described in the first part of this chapter and on the analysis of the improvement of the hearing ability after implantation of the artificial middle ear dealt with in the second part.

Structure of the Testing and Training Program

There were some individual differences among the 5 patients in hearing threshold before and after the operation and the daily use of the hearing ability. In each case, however, common items were found which had to be tested and trained in order for them to recover their hearing ability. This testing and training program set up based on clinical experience, with special emphasis on developing a method adapted to each patient's needs.

The rehabilitation program for the patients with MEIs is basically designed in the same way as that for patients with ordinary hearing aids. The program starts with (a) confirmation of the audiometric tests of the candidate for the implantation of the artificial middle ear, it includes such steps as (b) assessment of the patient's hearing ability for various types of sound sources before implantation; (c) prediction of the possibility of improvement after the implantation; (d) program to train hearing ability to achieve the predicted goal, and (e) comparison of the hearing ability before the implantation and after the training.

The improvement of hearing by use of the MEI will be assessed not only by the traditional pure-tone and speech audiometry before and after the operation, but also by the precise monitoring of the progress of the training. The rehabilitation program for patients with MEIs has many aspects in common with that of the cochlear implant [House, 1979; Maddox and Porter, 1983].

Confirmation of the Audiometric Tests of the MEI Candidate

As already has been discussed in part IV, the selection criteria of the MEI candidate are as follows:

(1) the ear to be operated on is not inflamed or the inflammation is under control, and the other ear has moderate hearing loss, causing difficulty in daily life;

(2) the bone-conduction hearing level in the ear to be operated on is less than 30 dB HL;

(3) there was no improvement after the previous operation, nor is any expected of middle ear reconstruction;

(4) sufficient vibratory sensation is observed during the preliminary operation.

At the present stage, only adults, whose bone growth is terminated, are considered for implantation. It will be beneficial to the patient if he has residual hearing in the high-frequency range so that he can utilize the sensitivity of the artificial middle ear up to 5 kHz. Prior to the implantation, it is also important that the tester but also the patient himself establish the maximum hearing ability achieved by using an optimally fitted ordinary hearing aid.

Assessment of the Patient's Hearing Ability before Implantation

The following items are to be recorded in detail regarding the characteristics of the patient's hearing ability for various types of sound source before implantation:

(1) analysis of the nature of perceptual confusion among vowels and consonants based on the response for Japanese syllables in traditional speech audiometry. Separation of the individual problems from the general ones caused by the characteristics of his hearing loss;

(2) inquiry about the patient's impression of the sounds caused by his hearing ability. This could be useful for selecting sound materials for training;

(3) preparation of the method of quantitative evaluation for the efficiency of transmission of speech information by finding the speech materials frequently used in his daily life.

Data which are necessary for preparing materials for training of hearing ability are as follows:

Data on the patient's own voice: items necessary for detailed analysis of the individual characteristics of the hearing ability are: (1) speech quality including sex, age, pitch (average fundamental frequency), loudness (average intensity level), tonal quality (average spectral inclination); (2) dialect including area (place of birth, marriage); phone (formant frequencies of the vowels, spectral and temporal characteristics of consonants), prosody (accent and intonation), vocabulary (peculiar words); (3) personal characteristics including education (major), vocation (field) and expression (frequently used phrases). These data can be obtained from the interview with the patients, recording of his speech, and acoustical analysis of the recorded speech with a sound level meter, pitch extractor and spectrograph.

Data on speech of other persons: in order to adjust the sensitivity of the artificial middle ear and to train the hearing ability to be suitable for objective speech, similar data on following speech are necessary: (1) speech of his family (spouse, children, parents and brothers/sisters); (2) speech of his colleagues, neighbors, relatives and friends. Check the persons among those who have to talk over the telephone.

Data on sound sources other than speech: the acoustic data on the following sounds which are frequently listened to or important in the patient's daily life are necessary in addition to the above speech data: (1) kind of music (songs, instruments, favorite pieces) and sounds found in his daily environment (indoor sounds, outdoor sounds, alarms, hobbies).

Prediction of Possibility of Improvement after the Implantation

It is impractical to connect directly the aided characteristics and the hearing ability for various kinds of sound sources, because many stages are considered to be intermediate between them. In order to relate them quantitatively, the characteristics of each of these stages should be taken into account. The intermediate stages are: adjustment of the electroacoustic sensitivity of the artificial middle ear for the hearing loss of each individual patient, the audible amplitude-frequency range which is determined by the sensitivity of the artificial middle ear, acoustical properties of objective sounds including speech and others, prediction of the theoretical limit of speech intelligibility and discrimination of the tonal quality of other sounds based on those characteristics, and the auditory training for the optimal use of the predicted limit.

Corrections for individual characteristics of objective speech involve the average amount of formant frequency shift for all types of vowels due to the difference of shape of the vocal tract of the speaker, the deviation in the average value of the fundamental frequency, and the deviation in the intensity of unvoiced sounds relative to the vowels. The individual acoustical properties of specific consonants are also taken into account in the prediction. Corrections for the effects of the nonacoustical factors such as individual differences in ability of language understanding at these stages are also necessary.

Combining all these characteristics at the various stages, the effects of the modification of aided characteristics can be related to the improvement of hearing ability achieved as the result of appropriate training.

Training of Hearing Ability to Achieve the Predicted Goal

A few days before the implantation of the artificial middle ear, a set of tests, in addition to the routine pure-tone and speech audiometry, is conducted taking into account the patient's hearing characteristics. These data, as well as those obtained during the operation, are used to detect the effect of the aided characteristics as sensitively as possible and to find what should be done to promote the optimal use of mechanical hearing.

When the patient starts using the MEI, about 10 days after the operation, the volume and tone controls of the outside-body unit are preset to the most comfortable level predicted for the speech sound with an intensity level of 60 to 70 dB SPL and readjusted based on the results of the test in quiet conditions in a sound-proof room in the hospital. At the same time, all the capabilities of the device are examined and demonstrated to the patient. A set of tests and training of hearing ability, which takes about 60 min including the routine pure-tone and speech audiometry, are conducted almost every day during the patient's stay in the hospital. The test and training materials include a list of words which require high-frequency components for their discrimination, and are supposed to become intelligible with the aided characteristics. Also included are some familiar sounds helping the patient to detect slight differences of tonal quality. At the same time, the patient is shown how to use the MEI under a noisy environment in the hospital. This step also includes guidance in the manipulation of the outside-body unit, such as on/off of power switch, adjustment of the volume dial, selection of tone control (buss cutoff), checking the battery and maintenance of the unit. If necessary, the tests and training sessions are repeated at intervals of 1–2 weeks after discharge from hospital.

Comparison of the Hearing Ability before the
Implantation and after the Training

The results of a series of tests undertaken before and after the implantation are used for the detailed evaluation of the improvement of the hearing ability in the process of the training using the MEI.

The items used for the comparison are the minimal audible threshold, the audible amplitude-frequency range (the uncomfortable level and most comfortable level), various aspects of tonal quality discrimination and speech intelligibility. Other items also considered are the intensity level of patient's own speech, the opinion of the patient on the advantages of using the MEI compared with his preimplantation status, the ordinary hearing aid, and the hearing in the other ear.

In the training process and in the evaluation, the use of the binaural effect in hearing various sounds, including speech in daily life, is considered as one of the most beneficial aspects of the implantation. This is the reason why the patients having residual hearing in the other ear comparable to the predicted aided characteristics for the implanted ear are selected for implantation. This will allow us to perform more precise and systematic perceptual tests using sound materials which are processed electroacoustically in various ways and presenting stimuli to both ears successively or simultaneously, in order to obtain qualitative descriptions of tonal quality of sound derived from mechanical hearing to which no persons other than the patients have a chance to listen to.

Shizuo Hiki, PhD, School of Human Science, Waseda University, Tokorozawa, Saitama 359 (Japan)

Adv. Audiol., vol. 4, pp. 149–159 (Karger, Basel 1988)

Efficacy of the Partially Implantable Middle Ear Implant in Middle and Inner Ear Disorders

Naoaki Yanagihara, Eizo Yamanaka, Hidemitsu Sato, Kiyofumi Gyo

Department of Otolaryngology, Ehime University School of Medicine, Ehime, Japan

Two types of middle ear implant (MEI), a totally implantable MEI (T-MEI) and a partially implantable MEI (P-MEI), have been developed. Direct stimulation of the stapes by an ossicular vibrator using a piezo-electric ceramic bimorph is the principal functional mechanism common to the both types of MEI. In addition to the ossicular vibrator, the T-MEI consists of an electret microphone, an electric amplifier with automatic gain control and a battery with an emergency cut-off switch. All the components coated by layers of biocompatible material are miniaturized enough to allow surgical implantation in the ear. The animal experiments as well as the tests in vitro indicated that clinical application of the T-MEI was theoretically and technically possible. However, we consider this clinical challenge to be still premature because of the following reasons: (1) we are not completely confident about the reliability and durability of the ossicular vibrator in the human ear, (2) the acoustic characteristics of the device cannot be adjusted externally when the grade of hearing impairment advances, and (3) a requirement for surgery in order to change the battery every 2 or 3 years may not be accepted by the patient. In view of the life of the device, the external adjustability of the acoustic characteristics and simplicity of the surgical procedure involved, we decided to apply the P-MEI preferentially to selected patients. On August 6, 1984, we successfully implanted the P-MEI for the first time to a 61-year-old male with mixed deafness of 55 dB due to intractable stenosis of the Eustachian tube and cholesterol granuloma. Encouraged by the success achieved by the first patient, we have implanted the device into 5 other patients over the past 4 months. This paper describes the efficacy of the P-MEI on the basis of our clinical experiences with these patients.

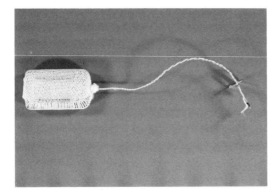

Fig. 1. Internal unit of a P-MEI

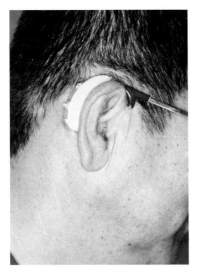

Fig. 2. External unit of a P-MEI

Components of the P-MEI

The P-MEI is composed of an internal and an external unit. The internal unit consists of the vibrator element made of a piezoelectric ceramic bimorph and an internal link coil (fig. 1). The element is 1.4 mm in width, 1.6 mm in thickness and 7.0 mm in length. The vibrator element is supported by an element designed by us, which allows precise contact be-

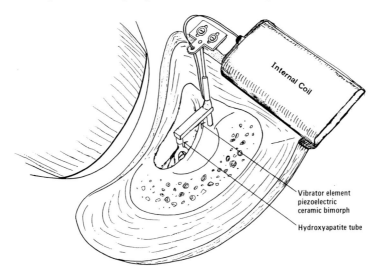

Vibrator element
piezoelectric
ceramic bimorph

Hydroxyapatite tube

Fig. 3. Surgical view after implanting the internal unit.

tween the tip of the element and the ossicle. The supporting installation consists of a holding plate and a supporting column. The holding plate is firmly fixed to the squamous portion of the temporal bone by stainless screws. The supporting column permits minute three-dimensional adjustments in the position of the vibrator element. Thus the tip of the vibrator is coupled with either the head of the stapes or the columella standing on the footplate of the stapes. The internal link coil placed under the retroauricular skin is activated from the outside by an outer link coil housed in a case together with the microphone, the amplifier and the battery, and is hung behind the auricle (fig. 2).

Surgical Procedure

Prior to retroauricular incision, a dummy of the external unit indicating the position of the external link coil is hung behind the auricle to determine where the internal link coil should be implanted. Through a retroauricular incision, a mastoidectomy and a posterior hypotympanotomy are performed in order to approach the stapes. Once the stapes is identified, a testing vibrator is attached to its head to measure the sensitivity of the vibrator. If the result indicates that the P-MEI will help the patient, the implantation of the P-MEI is finally decided at this moment and the surgical procedure initiated, as shown in figure 3.

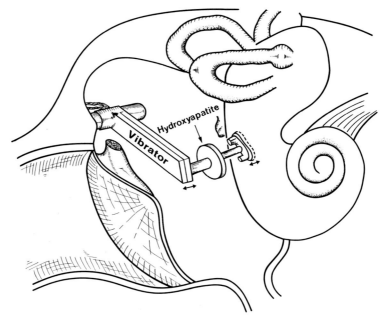

Fig. 4. Between the footplate and the tip of vibrator, a columella of hydroxyapatite is interposed where the superstructure of the stapes is missing.

A pocket for placing the internal link coil is created under the retroauricular skin by elevating the temporalis muscle and the thick connective tissue of the mastoid process and by drilling the squamous and mastoid portion of the temporal bone. The holding plate is firmly fixed in the most appropriate position of the zygomatic root with two screws, and the tip of the vibrator is carefully adjusted to connect with the stapes. Between the tip of the vibrator and the head of the stapes a tiny tube of hydroxyapatite is interposed. Thus the vibrator is properly connected to the head of the stapes. If the superstructure of the stapes is missing, a columella of hydroxyapatite is interposed between the footplate and the tip of the vibrator element (fig. 4). After incising the redundant temporalis muscle and the retroauricular connective tissue, the internal coil is inserted into the pocket. It is important to place the coil so as to secure the most efficient magnetic transmission between the outer and internal coils. Figure 3 shows the surgical view. Before closing the wound, the outer unit is placed on the skin over the internal link coil to determine whether the patient can hear through the device. Then the wound is closed.

Postoperative Treatment

The patient begins to use the device soon after healing of the retro-auricular wound. In order to determine the best volume adjustment and to learn how to use the outer unit, the patient needs several hours of training. Usually, no specific rehabilitation is necessary.

Indication

Considering the efficacy of the P-MEI, it could be applicable to patients with sensorineural hearing loss of moderate degree. However, for the present, we have limited utilization of the P-MEI to patients with mixed deafness due to middle ear disease since in such patients the advantages of the P-MEI are more definite. A patient who satisfies the following criteria would be an appropriate candidate for the P-MEI:

(1) average bone conduction in the speech frequencies of 500, 1,000, and 2,000 Hz not exceeding 40 dB;

(2) moderate to severe deafness in the contralateral ear.

(3) intraoperative vibratory hearing test proves that the hearing improvement afforded by the P-MEI is by far superior to that achieved by any reconstructive middle ear surgery.

Because of the excellent fidelity of sound transmission yielded by direct stimulation of the stapes and the good frequency characteristics of the vibrator, patients with impaired speech reception will be helped by the P-MEI. Needless to say, infection of the middle ear, if any, must be controlled prior to implantation of the device.

Clinical Results

Since the P-MEI was applied to the first patient, 2 years and 4 months ago, we have implanted into 5 other patients. Once the device was successfully implanted, it has continued to function and the patients have recovered very satisfactory hearing. Neither adverse effect on hearing nor foreign body tissue reaction has been noted.

All the 6 patients state that the sound quality provided by the P-MEI is indeed natural, clear, and easy to hear. Five of them had used conventional hearing aids previously. Therefore they were able to appreciate that the sound quality of the P-MEI was superior and easier to hear. They are agreed that the sound quality of the P-MEI is not at all artificial and that in this sense it is entirely different from that heard through a conventional hearing aid. The condensed case reports of each patients are described here.

Case 1. A 61-year-old male had suffered from bilateral otitis media since childhood. Seven years previously, in 1978, a tympanoplasty type III had been performed on the left ear. Since 1983, hearing impairment of the left ear had advanced to such a degree that he had encountered difficulty in his work. He consulted our university clinic on March 12, 1984. Microscopic inspection of the left ear and audiological examination indicated that no benefit would be derived from repeat tympanoplasty on the left ear. The right eardrum was somewhat yellowish, thick and retracted. Radiographies of the temporal bone revealed apparent inhibition of pneumatization. The patient strongly desired, if possible, to improve his hearing in the right ear.

On July 16, 1984, exploration of the right middle ear was carried out and cholesterin granuloma was found filling the mastoid and tympanic cavities. This granulation tissue was cleared. Fortunately, the stapes was found to be intact while the long process of the incus was eroded. A testing vibrator was coupled to the stapes and the sensitivity of the vibrator was assessed. The result suggested that the patient's hearing would be restored to a socially adequate level by using the P-MEI. The wound was then closed.

On August 6, 1984, the right ear was reexplored and the internal components were implanted. The postoperative course was uneventful and the patient began to use the device 1 week after the operation.

The audiogram in figure 5 shows the pre- and postoperative hearing. The postoperative hearing afforded by the P-MEI has been perfectly stable and the patient has had no difficulty in speech communication in his daily life.

Case 2. A 45-year-old male had suffered from bilateral otitis media since childhood. The right ear was operated on at the age of 8 years. In 1981, he consulted us complaining of bilateral deafness and was diagnosed as having cholesteatoma of the left ear and adhesive otitis media of the right ear. In 1982, staged tympanoplasties using the intact canal wall technique were carried out in both ears. The superstructures of the bilateral stapes were missing and hydroxyapatite ossicular columellas were used for reconstruction of sound conduction. Although hearing had been improved, the patient still had difficulty with his daily activites.

In July 1985, the internal components of the P-MEI were implanted in the left ear. The vibrator was coupled with a columella made of hydroxyapatite on the footplate. He was satisfied with his hearing improvement, shown in the audiogram in figure 6.

Case 3. A 45-year-old male had suffered from chronic otitis media of the bilateral ears since junior high school age. He consulted our university hospital in September 1984 and was diagnosed as having cholesteatoma of the left ear and cholesterol granuloma of the right ear. In December of 1984, a tympanoplasty type III using the intact

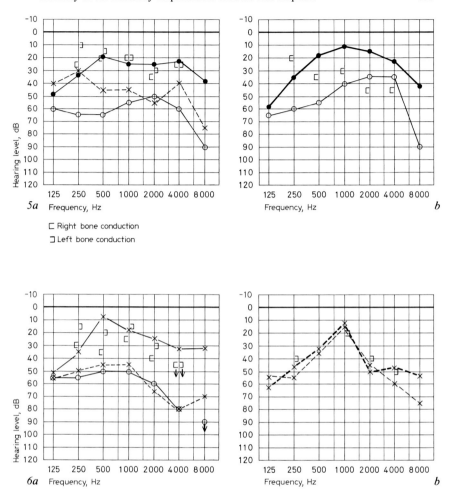

Fig. 5–10. Preoperative hearing levels and expected hearing threshold level afforded by the P-MEI *(a)* and postimplantation hearing threshold level afforded by the P-MEI and postoperative hearing level *(b)*. o—o = Right air conduction; x---x = left air conduction; x—x, •—• = expected hearing level afforded by the P-MEI; x_ _ _x, o_____o = postimplantation hearing level afforded by the P-MEI. *5* Patient 1. *a* Preoperative levels. *b* 2 years postoperatively. *6* Patient 2. *a* Preoperative levels. *b* 15 months postoperativeley. *7* Patient 3. *a* Preoperative levels. *b* 6 months postoperatively. *8* Patient 4. *a* Preoperative levels. *b* 5 months postoperatively. *9* Patient 5. *a* Preoperatively. *b* 4 months postoperatively. *10* Patient 6. *a* Preoperatively. *b* 1 month postoperatively.

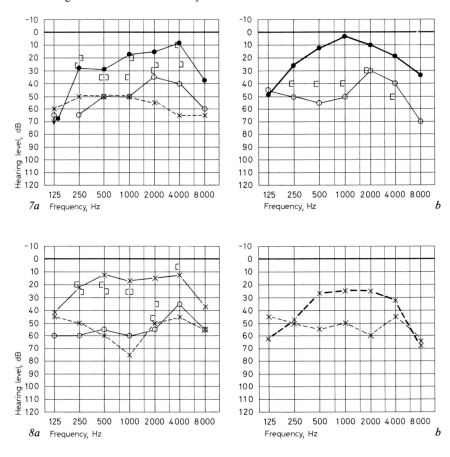

7a Frequency, Hz   b

8a Frequency, Hz   b

canal wall technique was performed on the left ear and in January of 1985, a tympano-plasty type III on the right ear. There was a large hidden cholesteatoma in the right ear and it was impossible to preserve the posterior ear canal. As is seen in the audiogram in figure 7a, he had difficulty in his work although an improvement of hearing was recognized postoperatively.

On December 13, 1985, the P-MEI was applied in the left ear. Since then, he has experienced no trouble caused by his hearing impairment. At the beginning of March 1986, he heavily struck his left temporal region while he was drunk. Since this accident, he had sensed fluctuations in the quality of hearing induced by the P-MEI. A temporal bone radiogram from Shuller's view revealed that one of the fixing screws was loose. On April 1, 1986, a revision operation was performed and the implanted components were removed without difficulty. No harmful tissue reaction was found and new inter-nal components were implanted. To prevent future shift of the holding plate, two screws of 7 mm diameter instead of 5 mm were used and firmly fixed to the holding plate.

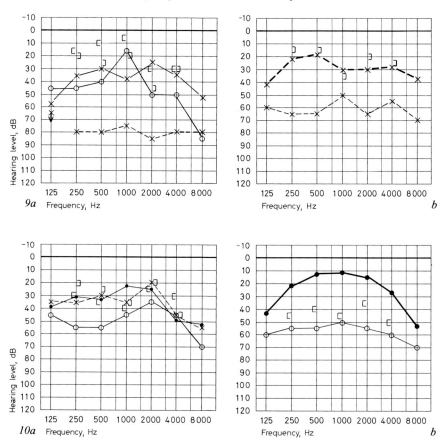

9a Frequency, Hz   b

10a Frequency, Hz   b

Postoperatively, his hearing has been restored to a stable state, the same as that before the accident. In figures 7a, b, his hearing before implantation of the P-MEI is compared with the postimplantation hearing.

Case 4. A 48-year-old male complained of bilateral deafness due to chronic otitis media since childhood. The left ear had been operated on at the age of 2, but the ear had always been draining. On inspection, granulation tisue filling the tympanic cavity was seen through a large defect in the eardrum. The right eardrum was atrophic and retracted.

   In June 1984, the left middle ear was explored and granulation tissue was cleaned. There were no auditory ossicles except for the footplate of the stapes. Because active inflammation was present, no reconstruction of the ossicular chain was attempted. Six months later, the tympanic cavity was reexplored. Although the aeration of the tympanic cavity was restored and a fine lining of healthy mucosa was seen, no satisfactory hearing restoration resulted from ossicular reconstruction using a hydroxyapatite ossicular prosthesis. During the operation, assessment of the vibratory hearing indicated that his hearing would be significantly improved by the P-MEI.

On June 24, 1986, the internal components of the P-MEI were implanted. The tip of the vibrator element was attached to a columella standing on the footplate. Ten days after the surgery, the patient began to use the device and was satisfied with the hearing facilitated by the P-MEI. In the audiogram in figures 8a, b, the pre- and postimplantation pure-tone hearing thresholds are displayed.

Case 5. A 58-year-old male had suffered from otitis media of bilateral ears in his childhood and noted profound deafness in his left ear. In September of 1984, he noted hearing impairment, pain and fullness in the right ear which was caused by cholesteatoma with labyrinthine fistula. By staged surgeries, the right hearing was saved but he had felt difficulty to understand conversation.

Otoscopic examination revealed a large perforation scar in the left eardrum without any signs of residual inflammation. Radiograms of the left temporal bone showed no finding of inflammation although pneumatization of the mastoid was moderately inhibited. A large gap between bone-conduction and air-conduction hearing levels suggested that an ossicular problem was involved (fig. 9a).

On July 15, 1986, the mastoid antrum was opened through a retroauricular incision. The incus and the superstructure of the stapes were missing although aeration and mucosal lining of the attic and atrum were nearly normal. The mobility of the footplate seemed to be inhibited by the surrounding scar tissue. A columella standing on the footplate was stimulated by the ossicular vibrator. As shown in figure 9b, the expected hearing level afforded by the P-MEI was about 30 dB, and restoration of hearing significant.

The length of the columella was adjusted so that the tip of the vibrator element touch the eardrum which might improve air-conduction hearing by virtue of a columella effect. Posteroperative hearing level is shown in figure 9b. The air-conduction hearing level was restored to the level expected by a usual ossiculoplasty. When he uses the P-MEI, his hearing is further improved beyond this level and close to normal hearing.

Case 6. A 56-year-old male had suffered from bilateral hearing impairment since his childhood and from repeated otitis media which was treated by myringotomies. No acute firing has occurred so far.

Both eardrums appeared to be somewhat yellowish, atrophic and retracted. The radiogram of the bilateral temporal bones showed inhibited pneumatization with slight thickening of the mucosa of the mastoid cells. Preoperative audiogram, as shown in figure 10a indicated bilateral mixed deafness of 50 dB in the right and 35 dB in the left ear.

Implantation of the P-MEI was attempted on September 30, 1986. The tympanic cavity and the antrum of moderate size as well were lined by smooth but thick mucosa and were well aerated. Although the continuity of the ossicular chain was preserved, its mobility was significantly limited. The stapes was surrounded by thick fibrous mucosa.

The incus and the head of the malleus were removed and a vibratory hearing test was done. As the result indicated that the P-MEI would restore satisfactory hearing, the implantation was carried out.

Postoperatively, his hearing level afforded by the P-MEI was close to normal at the speech frequencies (fig. 9b). He is using the P-MEI all day long, which helped his work greatly.

Discussion

A P-MEI using an ossicular vibrator of bimorph design was applied to 7 patient with mixed deafness of varying degree. The first patient proved that the device can function stably for an acceptably long period of time. All the patients have stated that the quality of sound was very natural, easy to hear and intelligible which, in turn, confirmed the advantages of direct oscillation of the stapes by the piezoelectric element. We emphasize that postimplantation hearing restoration cannot be surpassed by any type of usual reconstructive surgery.

Naoaki Yanagihara, MD, Department of Otolaryngology, Ehime University School of Medicine, Shigenobu-cho, Onsen-gun, Ehime 791-02 (Japan)

Adv. Audiol., vol. 4, pp. 160–166 (Karger, Basel 1988)

Implantation of Partially Implantable Middle Ear Implant and the Indication

Jun-Ichi Suzuki, Kazuoki Kodera, Hidemichi Ashikawa, Masakazu Suzuki

Department of Otolaryngology, Teikyo University School of Medicine, Tokyo, Japan

Indication of the Partially Implantable Middle Ear Implant

The indications of the partially implantable middle ear implant (P-MEI) are similar to those of tympanoplasty. As shown in part I, however, ears with mixed type hearing impairments and bone-conduction hearing thresholds between 20 and 40 dB are the best indication of the P-MEI.

In fact, the MEI is indicated only in patients with bilateral deafness. The ear to be selected for implantation is the ear with the worst hearing although, in most cases, we could get better results with the better hearing ear. This ear must have (1) a normal or normalized middle ear with no infections and with a pneumatized tympanum-attic-antrum cavity and (2) a near-normal inner ear with a usable speech discrimination score and a pure-tone bone conduction threshold between 20 and 40 dB.

If the patient has bilaterally mixed type deafness, determination of bone-conduction threshold of the ear with the worst hearing is frequently difficult and sometimes impossible. Speech audiometry, in such a case, may be a help in evaluating the inner ear function. Preoperative tests should also include the test using the piezoelectric vibrator and amplifier, etc., simulating the P-MEI. Although subjective evaluation is important, auditory brain stem response (ABR) is used also for the test for objective evaluation.

Method of Implantation of the P-MEI

Recent research on candidate patients revealed that the P-MEI was best indicated in two groups of cases: middle ear anomalies and chronic otitis media.

Both groups will be explored surgically. This is the first-step operation which is needed to prepare P-MEI implantation, the second step, as described in the case reports in the next section. The authors are using the method reconstructing but not preserving the posterior canal wall, as is explained in the following section.

Preparatory or First-Stage Operation for P-MEI Implantation

Patients with middle ear anomalies and/or microtia with atresia of the auditory canal and pure-tone bone-conduction thresholds between 20 and 40 dB are the candidates. In middle ear anomaly, the ossicles, especially the stapes, are examined. In microtia with atresia, in addition to exploring the ossicles and the stapes, the external canal, the attic and the antrum are reconstructed so as to be convenient for MEI implantation which will be conducted in about 6–12 months later.

Patients with chronic otitis media and/or cholesteatomatous otitis media are frequently the candidates for MEI. Cases with chronic or cholesteatomatous otitis media with pure-tone bone-conduction thresholds below 20 dB are the best candidates for tympanoplasty. Those who have bone-conduction thresholds between 20 and 40 dB are the best candidates for P-MEI implantation.

In this preparatory operation, the pathology is removed, the perforated eardrum is closed, and the whole middle ear cavity, including the attic and the antrum, is reconstructed to restore normal pneumatization and normal mucosal lining in the cavity. In 6–12 months, the whole middle ear cavity is usually normalized and becomes ready for P-MEI implantation. The stapes, or at least the stapes footplate, is inspected to make sure it is movable. A small or large opening is made in the antrum-attic wall depending on the pathology in these cavities. In cholesteatoma, the opening has to be sufficiently large to eradicate the cholesteatoma.

The antrum-attic wall, which is actually the canal wall, will be reconstructed by closing the opening with a bone plate taken from the temporal bone cortex (fig. 1). The transplanted bone plate survives by being covered with well-vascularized pedicles of periost and fascia. The whole

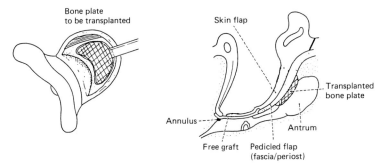

Fig. 1. Preparatory operation for P-MEI implantation. Posterior canal wall is reconstructed with a bone plate which is taken from the temporal bone cortex, and by covering the bone plate with pedicled flaps and the canal wall skin.

middle ear cavity is reconstructed and will be normalized in 6–12 months postoperatively and will be ready for P-MEI implantation.

Implantation or Second-Stage Operation for P-MEI Implantation

The second-stage operation will be conducted in 6–12 or more months after the first operation. The middle ear air space has to be checked, especially in cases of chronic otitis media. A couple of years may be needed until normalization of the cavity is completed. The best and easiest way is to use CT, which clearly shows air content in the Eustachian tube, tympanum, attic and antrum. The air in the attic-antrum, which is a good indication of normalization, is indispensable for safe and successful implantation of the P-MEI.

The second operation is performed under local anesthesia in order to make the hearing test during surgery possible. The skin incision for the first-stage operation is along the superior-posterior margin of the helix insertion (fig. 2a, *1). The skin incision for the second-stage operation should be largely posterior-superior to the helix insertion, as shown in figure 2a, *2. Temporal bone surface in the retroauricular area is widely drilled and a shallow dent is made just to hold the internal induction coil. The place to hold the internal coil should be carefully determined to meet best with the external coil (fig. 2a, 3). The correspondence of the external and internal coils is not too critical but still important (fig. 2b).

The skin along the posterior ear canal wall is elevated, and the antrum-attic wall is opened in the area, which is convenient for setting both the vibrator holder and the vibrator (fig. 3).

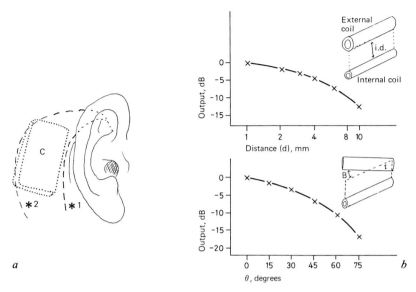

Fig. 2. Skin incision and implantation of the internal induction coil. *a* Skin incision for the first-stage (*1) and the second stage operation (*2). C = Internal induction coil. *b* The internal induction coil is to be placed properly to function together with the external induction coil in the best efficiency. Refer to these experimental data.

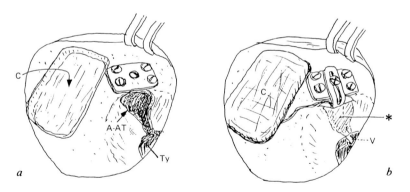

Fig. 3. Implantation of vibrator and internal induction coil into the right temporal bone. *a* Before implantation, showing the spaces for the vibrator holder in the antrum-attic (A-AT) and the dent for the coil (C). Ty = tympanum. *b* After implantation: the internal coil is placed in the dent and the vibrator holder and vibrator (V), in the attic-antrum. The canal wall is then closed by a bone or a cartilage plate (*).

A dummy vibrator holder is first used for the explorations. The real vibrator holder which is partly bendable is then adjusted exactly according to the dummy, and then firmly fixed to the temporal bone cortex with four screws. The vibrator tip is lightly touched on the stapes head or on the footplate without any positive or negative pressure. These two maneuvers to fix the vibrator holder and the vibrator have to be done simultaneously. The function of the P-MEI is then tested by coupling the internal and the external induction coils. The hearing test is carefully conducted to conclude the implantation. The internal induction coil is then placed in the shallow dent and fixed by suturing the soft tissues.

Since the implantation is performed in a normal or normalized middle ear, postoperative recovery should be fast and uncomplicated. Postoperative hearing tests are repeated during the recovery course. Within 10–14 days after surgery, the external part of the P-MEI can be held behind the ear as long as the patients wishes.

Case Reports on P-MEI Implantation

Two cases are reported: one, a case of microtia with atresia, and another, a case of chronic otitis media.

Case 1. This 33-year-old male (H. H.) had had bilaterally impaired hearing since childhood, due to chronic otitis media on the right and microtia with atresia on the left. Both ears had already been operated on several years ago in another hospital. His left ear was operated on again in our hospital and type I tympanoplasty improved his hearing to some extent. The audiograms before and after the tympanoplasty on the left ear are shon in figure 4 a.

Because the patient wanted to have further hearing improvement, implantation of the P-MEI was attempted in the right abnormal ear on July 22, 1985. Fortunately, for the P-MEI implantation, the previous operation in the other hospital had made the eardrum laterally positioned, and the middle ear cavity was found fairly normalized and substantially spacious, convenient for holding the vibrator holders. The stapes was hardly visible in the depth, but, fortunately again, the incus was connected to the stapes and movable. The vibrator tip was tentatively placed on the incus body, and the hearing then showed remarkable improvement. The P-MEI was implanted with the vibrator tip on the incus body. The results of the postoperative hearing tests are shown in figure 4b, c. The speech audiogram also showed remarkable improvement.

As shown in figure 4 c, the implanted ear showed a score a little better than that of the right ear also on the speech discrimination test. The speech discrimination score then showed gradual improvement during the early postoperative days. The explanation of this 'gradual improvement in speech discrimination' may be found in the fact that the ear had hardly been used for the 33 years of the patient's life.

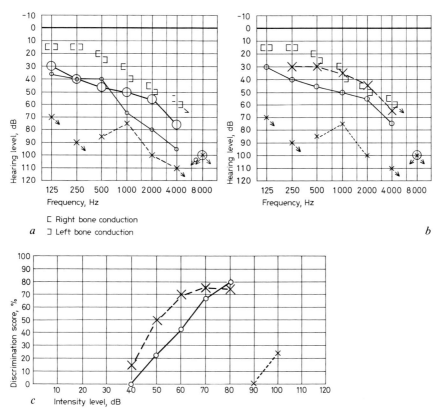

C Right bone conduction
a   ⅃ Left bone conduction   b

Fig. 4. Case 1. Hearing improvement by tympanoplasty and P-MEI implantation. *a* Pure-tone audiogram of the right ear before (o——o) and after (O——O) type 1 tympanoplasty. *b* Pure-tone audiogram of the left ear with MEI (X–––X) and without MEI (x-----x). *c* Speech audiogram of the left ear with MEI (X–––X) and without MEI (x-----x), and that of the right ear operated on by tympanoplasty (O——O).

As may be seen from the postoperative hearing test results, although the hearing improved by the P-MEI was better than the hearing on the other side, the patient wanted a little more improvement. The external part of the P-MEI could be intensified by about 10 dB. This increase in gain of the P-MEI gave the patient some satisfaction.

He has been observed and tested for 16 months until now. He appeared to be happy also with the other ear, which was operated on with tympanoplasty in our hospital, and showed some hearing improvement during the period of observation.

Case 2. This 59-year-old male (Y. M.) had bilateral chronic otitis media when he visited our clinic. Type I tympanoplasty was conducted on both ears. The hearing was improved postoperatively but was not sufficient for his daily life (fig. 5 a). As may be seen in the audiogram, his hearing exactly fitted the indication of P-MEI implantation.

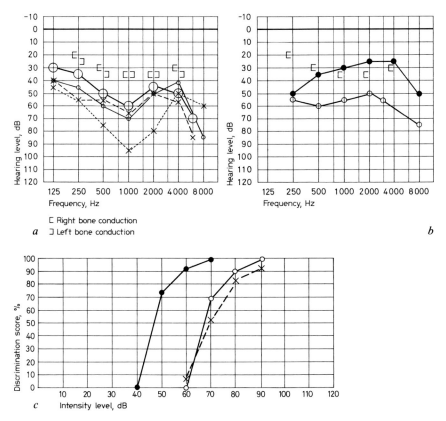

C Right bone conduction
a   ⅃ Left bone conduction   b

Fig. 5. Hearing improvement by tympanoplasty and P-MEI implantation. *a* Pure-tone audiogram before (o——o, x-----x) and after (O——O, X----X) type 1 tympanoplasty on both ears. *b* Pure-tone audiogram of the right ear with P-MEI (●——●) and without P-MEI (O——O). *c* Speech audiograms of the right ear with P-MEI (●——●) and without P-MEI (O——O) and of the left ear (X----X).

On January 13, 1986, a P-MEI was implanted to the right ear which was then the better hearing ear. The hearing obtained with the P-MEI in this ear is shown in figure 5b, c. Both pure-tone and speech perceptions were improved.

Since then he has been continuously using the MEI with high satisfaction. The hearing level in the implanted ear has not shown any change during the last 12 months. He has been enjoying the pure and clear speech sounds conveyed by the P-MEI. Actually, he is awaiting another implantation to the other side – next time with the totally implantable MEI.

Jun-Ichi Suzuki, MD, Department of Otolaryngology, Teikyo University School of Medicine, Itabashi-ku, Tokyo 173 (Japan)

Adv. Audiol., vol. 4, pp. 167–169 (Karger, Basel 1988)

Publication List[1]

1   Araki, H.; Suzuki, K.; Ohno, T.: The efficacy of a piezoelectric ceramic vibrator for the implantable hearing aid. Proceedings for the Spring Meeting, No. 1, pp. 157–158 (Acoust, Soc. Jpn., Tokyo 1981).

2   Araki, H.; Honma, A.; Suzuki, K.: The microphone and the vibrator for an implantable hearing aid, their construction and evaluation. Technical report of the hearing research group, No. H–83–44, pp. 1–7 (Acoust. Soc. Jpn., Tokyo 1983).

3   Berger, K. W.: The hearing aid, its operation and development. Nat. H. A. Soc. (1970).

4   Blood, G. W.: The hearing aid 'effect', H. A. J. 28: 12 (1977).

5   Cook, R. O.; Royster, L. H.; Thomas, W. G.; Prazma, J.; Hickham, J.: A flexure mode piezoelectric transducer for driving the ossicular chain of research animals. J. acoust. Soc. Am. 54: 293 (1973).

6   Cook, R. O.; Hamm, C. W.; Thomas, W. G.; Royster, L. H.: Comparison of acoustically coupled and mechanically coupled speech. Audiology 20: 516–529 (1981).

7   Elbrond, O.; Elpern, B. S.: Reconstruction of ossicular chain in incus defects. An experimental study. Archs Otolar. 82: 603–608 (1965).

8   Fukuyama, K.; Yamamoto, T.; Masaike, H.; Suzuki, J.; Kodera, K.: Composition and specification of the implantable hearing aids. Technical report of the hearing research group, No. H–83–46, pp. 1–8 (Acoust. Soc. Jpn., Tokyo 1983).

9   Funai, H.; Funasaka, S.; Matayoshi, M.: Development of an electromagnetic transducer for direct oscillation of the middle ear ossicles. Audiol. Jpn. 23: 79–84 (1980).

10 Fredrickson, J. M.; Tomlinson, D. R.; Davis, E. R.: Evaluation of an electromagnetic implantable hearing aid. Can. J. Otolaryngol. 2: 54–62 (1973).

11 Glorig, A.; Moushegian, G.; Bringewald, P. R.; Rupert, A. L.; Gerken, G. M.: Letters to the editor. J. acoust. Soc. Am. 52: 694–696 (1972).

12 Goode, R. L.: An implantable hearing aid. Trans. Am. Acad. Ophthal. Oto-lar. 74: 128–139 (1970).

13 Goode, R. L.: Toward an implantable hearing aid. H. A. J. 28: 10 (1975).

14 Goode, R. L.: Implantable hearing aid may be ready in five years. Audecibel 26: 68 (1977).

[1] References for the papers from Japan are listed.

15 Guinan, J. J., Jr.; Peake, W. T.: Middle ear characteristics of anesthetized cats. J. acoust. Soc. Am. *41*: 1237–1261 (1967).

16 Gyo, K.; Yanagihara, N.; Araki, H.: The hearing perception by the piezoelectric ceramic vibrator during a tympanoplasty operation. Audiol. Jpn. *25*: 429–430 (1982).

17 Gyo, K.; Yanagihara,N.; Hiki, S.: The subjective clinical evaluation of the vibrator for the implantable hearing aid. Technical report of the hearing research group, No. H–83–45, pp. 1–6 (Acoust. Soc. Jpn., Tokyo 1983).

18 Gyo, K.; Aritomo, H.; Goode, R. L.: Measurement of the ossicular vibration ratio in human temporal bones by use of a video-measuring system. Acta oto-lar. (in press).

19 Gyo, K.; Goode, R. L.; Miller, G.: Experimental study of stapes vibration produced by the output transducer of an implantable hearing aid. Am. J. Otol. *82*: 603–608 (1987).

20 Hough, J.; Vernon, J.; Johnson, B.; Dormer, K.; Himelick, T.: Experiences with implantable hearing devices and a presentation of a new device. Annls Oto-lar. *95*: 60–65 (1986).

21 House, W.; Berliner, K.; Eisenberg, L.: Present status and future directions of the Ear Research Institute cochlear implant program. Acta oto-lar. *87*: 170–184 (1979).

22 Kodera, K.; Yamane, H.; Suzuki, K.; Araki, H.: the efficacy of a piezoelectric ceramic vibrator for the implantable hearing aid. Jpn. J. artif. Organs *10*: 524–527 (1981).

23 Kodera, K.; Suzuki, J.; The medical evaluation of input and output transducer for the implantable hearing aid. Technical report of the hearing research group, No. H-81-47, pp. 1–6 (Acoust. Soc. Jpn., Tokyo 1981).

24 Levitt, H: Hearing aids: prescription, selection, evaluation, App.: The phonograph, telephone, hearing aids, and the development of speech audiometry; in Levitt, Pickett, Houde, Sensory aids for the hearing impaired, pp. 29–38 (IEEE Press, New York 1980).

25 Maddox, H.; Porter, T.: Who is a candidate for cochlear implantation? In Arenberg, Symposium on Inner Ear Surgery. Otolaryngol. Clin. North Am. *16*: 249–255 (1983).

26 Ministry of International Trade and Industry Japan: R and D on medical and welfare apparatus technology, p. 13 (AIST, Tokyo 1986).

27 Northern, J. I.: The current status of implantable hearing aid. H. A. J. *26*: 14–43 (1973).

28 Nunley, J. A.; Agnew, J.; Smith, C. L.: A new design for an implantable hearing aid. ISA BM *76313*: 69–72 (1976).

29 Ohno, T.: The implantable hearing aid. Part I. Audecibel *33*: 28–30 (1984).

30 Ohno, T.: The implantable hearing aid. Part II. Audecibel *34*: 22–24 (1985).

31 Pascoe, D.: Clinical implications of nonverbal methods of hearing aid selection and fitting. Semin. Speech, Language and Hearing *1*: 217–229 (1980).

32 Pollack, M. C.: Amplification for the hearing-impaired (Grune & Stratton, New York 1980).

33 Shaw, E. A. G.: The sound pressure transformation from the free-field to the ear drum, No. 34, pp. 745 (Acoust. Soc. Am., 1962).

34 Shaw, E. A. G.: Transformation of sound pressure from the free field to the ear drum in the horizontal plane. J. acoust. Soc. Am. *56:* 1848–1861 (1974).

35 Shono, H.; Takinishi, K.; Suzuki, K.; Fukuyama, K.; Suzuki, J.; Ikeda, H.: Some composition of the implantable hearing aid and its functions. Jpn. J. artif. Organs *11:* 516–519 (1982).

36 Shono, H.; Takinishi, K.; Ikeda, H., et al.: The implantable hearing aid. Final technical report, pp. 22–45, 78–103 (Technology Research Association of Medical and Welfare Appartus, Tokyo 1983).

37 Shono, H.; Takinishi, K.; Ikeda, H., et al.: The implantable hearing aid. Final technical report, pp. 90–97 (Technology Research Association of Medical and Welfare Apparatus, Tokyo 1983).

38 Suzuki, J.: On the project of implantable artificial middle ear. Technical report of the hearing research group, No. H-65-5, pp. 1–7 (Acoust. Soc. Jpn., Tokyo 1979).

39 Suzuki, J.; Kodera, K.: Problems with hearing aids at use and the project of implantable artificial middle ear. J. Acoust. Soc. Jpn. *35:* 43–47 (1979).

40 Suzuki, J.; Shono, H.; Ikeda, H.: Problems and solutions in the implantation and acoustic characteristics of an implantable artificial middle ear. Jpn. J. artif. Organs *9:* 495–498 (1980).

41 Suzuki, J.; Toriyama, M.; Hiki, S.: Implantable artificial middle ear. Prospects of its technological development. J. acoust. Soc. Jpn. *36:* 108–109 (1980).

42 Suzuki, J.: Various approaches for the improvement of hearing; in Pfaltz, Adv. Oto-Rhino-Laryng, vol. 29, pp. 194–198 (Karger, Basel 1983).

43 Suzuki, J.; Kodera, K.; Yanagihara, N.: Evaluation of middle-ear implant. A six-month observation in cats. Acta oto-lar. *95:* 646–650 (1983).

44 Suzuki, J.; Yanagihara, N.: Middle ear implant – implantable hearing aid. Art.-M. A. News *4:* 10–13 (1983).

45 Suzuki, J.: New dimensions in otology, tympanoplasty and middle ear implants; in Myers, New dimensions in otorhinolaryngology – head and neck surgery, No. 1, pp. 39–42 (Elsevier Scientific, Amsterdam 1985).

46 Suzuki, J.; Kodera, K.; Yanagihara, N.: Middle ear implant for humans. Acta oto-lar. *99:* 313–317 (1985).

47 Suzuki, J.-I.; Yanagihara, N.; Kadera, K.: The partially implantable middle ear implant, case reports. Adv. Oto-Rhino-Laryng. *37:* 178–184 (Karger, Basel 1987).

48 Vernon, J.; Brummet, R.; Denniston, R.; Doyle, P.: Evaluation of an implantable type hearing aid by means of cochlear potentials. Volta Rev. *74:* 20–29 (1972).

49 Vernon, J.: The implantable hearing instrument. Hearing Instruments *27:* 10–12 (1976).

50 Watanabe, T.: Responses of primary auditory neurons to electromagnetic driving of the ear drum. Jap. J. Physiol. *15:* 92–100 (1965).

51 Wilpizeski, C.; Spector, M.: A simple implantable electromechanical middle ear. Trans. Penns. Acad. Ophthal. Otol. *32:* 41–46 (1979).

52 Yanagihara, N.; Gyo, K.; Suzuki, K.; Araki, H.: Perception of sound through direct oscillation of the stapes using a piezoelectric ceramic bimorph. Ann. Otol. *92:* 223–227 (1983).

53 Yanagihara, N.; Suzuki, J.; Gyo, K.; Syono, H.; Ikeda, H.; Development of an implantable hearing aid using a piezoelectric vibrator of bimorph design. State of the art. Am. Acad. Otolaryng. *92:* 706–712 (1984).

Subject Index